Chekhov's Lie

Also by Harold L. Klawans, M.D.

Chekhov's Lie

Harold L. Klawans, M.D.

To Katie

With best wishes

Harold

demos vermande ❖

A few of the neuroscientists depicted in this novel, Bill Landau and David Garron, are real people and are depicted as such. This is, however, a novel, a work of fiction. All other characters are fictitious and all other names are used fictitiously. Except for base-ball players other than Marty Bloom. Bloom is a product of my imagination and should not be confused with any baseball player, living or dead. The other baseball players were all real.

Library of Congress Cataloging-in-Publication Data

Klawans, Harold L.
    Chekhov's lie / Harold L. Klawans.
      p. cm.
    ISBN 1-888799-12-9
    I. Title.
PS3561.L336C48   1997
813'.54—dc21   97-25498
                                           CIP

Made in the United States of America

For David, Dannie, Bill, and all those who have helped make a life in literature and medicine possible for me, and to Barbara, who has helped me live that life to the fullest.

Acknowledgments

I am indebted to two individuals who were of great help to me in editing this book: Suzanne Poirier of the University of Illinois College of Medicine and editor-in-chief of *Literature and Medicine,* and Joan Wolk of Demos Vermande. Roger's attitude toward editors should not be confused with my high regard for all the assistance I have received from the thoughtful and helpful suggestions of these two editors. At times I was too stubborn to accept their judgments, but I will be the one who has to live with and reread the results.

Chekhov's Lie

July

"Do you know my name?" I asked the patient. I did not expect Mr. Hayes to recall my name. He had been my patient for only a few days. We had met only a couple of times. And he had severe memory difficulties that we thought would turn out to be due to Alzheimer's disease.

He looked at me quizzically, as if he was trying to summon whatever ability to recall names that remained functioning. "Would it help me if I did?" he finally replied.

"No," I admitted, "probably not."

Harold L. Klawans
Newton's Madness

July 1—9 A.M.

Dear Rob,

I find it hard to believe that we have not talked, written, or communicated with each other at all in the last twenty-nine years. That one year we spent together as interns does not seem like yesterday to me. It's at least one entire lifetime ago; yet how did we lose all contact? We would both have bet against that ever happening. But it did. How did you ever wind up in obstetrics and gynecology? I thought you were going to be an internist. That seemed to be you. That shows what little insight we had into one another back then, but who had time for insight into each other? We had all we could do to keep the patients alive until our shift was over. Interns and their perspectives have unfortunately not progressed very far.

And now you want to become a writer, an AUTHOR! I'm sure your specialty will give you a somewhat peculiar, if not unique, viewpoint. I once toyed with writing a play that opened with the heroine undergoing a pelvic examination. All done discreetly, of course, behind a curtain, with light coming from behind her. A silhouette of her with legs in the stirrups. And the vaginal speculum descending. Its size exaggerated by the back lighting. A great opening. Calculated to get everyone's attention. It was all downhill from there. So, yes, there is some advice I'd like to pass along to you.

First, instead of killing all the lawyers, the fantasy of all those other physicians, let's start by destroying some of the myths that surround your fantasy of becoming a physician-writer, a part of that time-honored tradition of Conan Doyle, Anton Chekhov, and Arthur Schnitzler. William Carlos Williams. And today Oliver Sacks. They are myths that I once believed. But no more.

Foremost is Chekhov's own myth. Our beloved Chekhov, the first modern physician who really made it as a writer, the father of us all. Well, I've got news for you, Rob. You are sitting down, I hope. Good ol' Chekhov lied to us and he also undoubtedly lied to himself. From the point of view of scientists, and we are all that, medical scientists, true, but scientists by training, from that viewpoint, all writers lie. Whatever else they are, observers, commentators, speculators, fantasists, writers are neither scientists nor reporters. The problem is we are more likely to believe authors than we are to believe either scientists or reporters. After all, both scientists and reporters can be easily misled by erroneous data, by mistaken witnesses, but writers, real authors, are seekers of the real truth. An example. Kafka. Compare *The Metamorphosis* with any paper in your field published the same year. Any one? Your pick. Can you even cite a paper written seven decades ago that still has some truth in it? But Chekhov lied to me and to you. Perhaps he was kidding us. He couldn't have really believed what he wrote. Certainly no modern reader can take him seriously. His lie? His famous remark that juggling his two careers, medicine and writing, was like juggling a wife and a mistress and that neither the former nor the latter suffered a bit from his juggling act. He went on to write that he felt more contented and more satisfied because he had two professions, not one, both a wife and a mistress. Medicine he called his lawful wife, and literature, his mistress. When he grew weary of one, he passed the night with the other. "This may seem disorderly," he continued, "but it is not dull, and besides, neither of them suffers because of my infidelity." No wife or mistress, modern or not, would buy that for an instant, but it is quoted over and over again, passed on from man to man, from one physician-writer to the next. No more. Not from me to you. That lie stops here.

I've got news for you: writing, good writing, requires intense, if not libidinal, effort. Like giving proper attention to your wife. If you put that energy into writing, something else will have to suffer from not receiving that effort, that intensity, that portion of your libidinal energy. Chekhov, I remind you, was not married at the time he tried juggling his two careers. He got married years after he'd given up practicing medicine to devote all his time and energy to writing. So, you ask, has my professional life as a physician suffered by my pursuing a second career? Of course it has. That was inevitable, Rob. Oh, I could be like Chekhov and point out that I see more patients now than I ever did. Or that I listen to my patients more closely than I did in the past. I am now more likely to hear what they are telling me, not just the words they are saying, but the subtext in addition. They are, after all, one of my primary sources. My inspiration. Or . . . . But why should I lie to you? I have tried to give up lying to myself. Unlike Chekhov. His lie may well have been his own delusion. There is a difference. Self-delusion must also go. Lying to yourself is out. Good advice for both the writer and the scientist in both you and me. The answer, my old friend, is "yes." At one time I sustained the classic academic career that encompassed teaching, patient care, clinical research, and basic science research. I ran a laboratory that was on the cutting edge of whatever research we were doing. I competed successfully for federal grants. I wrote major research papers. Real science. They are still quoted today, twenty years later. Never fear, they won't live as long as *The Metamorphosis*. I am not destined to become an eponym. But they have had a good run. I did some important research. I produced pivotal papers. No more. I still teach as much as I ever did and just as effectively, I think. I still do as much clinical research as ever. You've already heard about my patients. But I haven't been inside "my" lab in a decade. So much for the cutting edge, Rob. That's all history. So give up Chekhov's myth. Something will have to go when you acquire your new mistress. If she is anything more than just a one-night stand, your relationship to your wife will change. She'll know and you'll know. So much for that fantasy.

Once you get started, your professional associates, both those who are friends and those who aren't, especially those who aren't, will tell you that finding the time to write must be impossible. Their implication is that you must be neglecting your patients. Did any man ever chastise a wayward friend for neglecting his wife? Or am I pushing the analogy too far? You're a busy physician. You have an office full of patients. Forget it, Rob, there isn't any time. You've probably already heard the litany from fellow physicians as they debate each detail of some obscure football game between two college teams playing in some bowl game you didn't know existed. The Cherry Bowl. The Salad Bowl. The Toilet Bowl. Whatever. The problem is not finding the time, the question is using the time. Physicians we both know, ones with whom we interned, have season tickets to both the Chicago Bulls and the Chicago Blackhawks. Together, including the play-offs, that's about one hundred home games per year—not counting the Bears, the Cubs, or the White Sox. And the equal number of road games that are on TV. Just the home games. One hundred home games at four hours per game including travel time and all those TV time-outs, that's four hundred hours.

Four hundred hours! Think of that amount of free time, Rob. In four hundred hours I can write a novel. Two drafts. No one asks that sports fan where he finds the time to go to all those games. This letter, once started, took me less time than a Bulls game. If there had been an overtime, the game would have taken longer. And undoubtedly been more exciting.

So where is that time? I write in the mornings, Rob. William Carlos Williams wrote in the evenings and between patients. Whenever he could find a couple of minutes. Williams kept his typewriter in his office desk. All he needed to do was to pull up the leaf of his desk and he was ready to go. He would type away at top speed. If a patient came in while he was in the middle of a sentence, he'd put away his typewriter and he was once again a physician. When the patient left, the typewriter and the writer reemerged simultaneously. Today, with word processing on your own PC, that would be even easier. It's not a practice I recommend. All I do between patients is jot down notes, comments, quotes, ideas. Not full-fledged drafts.

I also try to arrange each of my weeks so that I can devote most of Sunday morning to rewriting, to revising whatever I tried to put together earlier in the week. I get up at five thirty or so, make a pot of coffee, and work until noon. Then once every three months I block out an entire weekend and revise everything I've done in those three months. Just like any other business. It's my literary quarterly report. Whenever I'm finishing a book I have a fantasy of a week of Sunday mornings to get things really right. My idea of paradise is a month of Sundays. More than that would require the coming of the Messiah. Somehow I manage without Him. This weekend I am devoting my morning to you. Don't feel guilty. Or honored. I have my motives. Writers always do.

You, I assume, want to write a novel. Most physicians start off with novels. That's probably because we're basically conservative. We still think in terms of novels. And we're also just a bit grandiose. You could do a short story or two before your first novel. It wouldn't hurt. Unfortunately, the great American screenplay is where the money is. Or perhaps the great American sit-com. Or is that an oxymoron?

It will come as a surprise to some people, but the odds are that you did not go to medical school to become a writer. I sure as hell know that I didn't. It's one of those universal assumptions. You've started to write, ergo you always wanted to be a writer. Why else would you want to become a writer now? If you took up golf, no one would assume that you always wanted to be a golf pro. I started my first novel because I just wanted to see if I could do it. I've always been an avid reader of novels. You must remember that much about me. Even during my internship, I always had at least one nonmedical book on me at all times. They were usually novels. Novels of all sorts from Ambler to Yourcenaur. I can't think of any Z's right now. Could I write one? Once I asked myself the question, I had to find out. Could I write a real novel? One with a beginning, a middle, and an end. And characters. And plot. And location. And tone. And purpose. Just like a real writer. Maybe even with a style of writing. Could I do that? There was only one way to find out.

Then I realized that there was something I wanted to write about— teaching the art of diagnosis. A lot of things have changed since we were interns, but over the last couple of decades the one constant in my life has been teaching. It is a passion of mine. My first Chekhovian mistress. I worked at it passionately. Teaching medical students how to understand a patient's story. Teaching residents how to think about sick people. I didn't write my first book because I'd always needed to write, to express myself, to become a published author. That all came later. I wrote my first novel over a period of three months in 1975. When it was completed, I made ten copies of it and gave them to my friends and family and then put the original in the basement and redirected my libido back to my laboratory. Five years later I submitted that draft to a publisher who accepted it. It was then, as I rewrote it, that I discovered how much I loved writing, nonmedical writing, and my life as an author began.

So, no, Rob, I didn't always need to be a writer. Expression was not always the need of my soul. It just is now and forever.

Others will tell you that it's impossible to combine writing with the practice of medicine. That two careers is one career too many. What bunk! Most writers have two careers for much of their lives, many for all their lives. Those "day jobs" are the real means of subsistence for writers, actors, composers, painters, poets, and virtually every other "creative artist." The fact is that of all those who aspire to success as writers physicians have pretty much the best day jobs. You probably never thought about it like that. Most people haven't. Our jobs are demanding; there's no question about that. But so is waiting on tables. If you don't believe me, Rob, try it yourself. And then remember that when you give your next tip. Fifteen percent. Is that all? And practicing medicine pays a hell of a lot better. Your biggest conflict will not be between practicing medicine and writing, in terms of energy or time. The biggest conflict will be money. A lot of other physicians have told me of their need to write. More than you might imagine. But they just couldn't cut down on their practice. They couldn't afford it. Couldn't? Give me a break. And then they drive off in a Porsche or a Jaguar. They evoke little sympathy from me. It is *not* just the practice of medicine with which the need to write will compete. It's the standard of affluence that comes with practicing medicine, that's the real competition.

And keep this one fact in mind, you don't write to make money. To make money you do another hysterectomy, or cover another hospital, or extend your office hours, or open a sleep lab. You write because you want to write, because you need to write. And I know you, Rob; you went into medicine for the same reasons I did. You wanted to take care of sick people. Good. You can still do that. And do that very well.

Perhaps not for quite as many hours a week. Big deal. You don't really need that condo in Aspen, do you? Or that new Porsche? Or are you still into Corvettes?

And one of the things you wrote in your letter is all backwards. I know you believe it, but the mere fact that you think you communicate well with your patients will not make you a good writer. Being a "people person" is not what writing is all about. In a way that's the most dangerous trap of all. It's not an oxymoron; it's an absolute contradiction in terms. Good writing must communicate something from the author to the reader, but that end point depends upon both the author and the reader and it is one over which the author has no control once the word is set on the page. Communication is the essence of good writing but the most significant element in that communication is self-communication. That has little if anything to do with being a "people person." Writing is a solitary occupation. Perhaps the most solitary occupation of all. An artist can have a model. A composer, some instrumentalist or other. Even a whole quartet. But a writer has a blank piece of paper and a pen. Or the blank screen of his monitor. Take your pick. The process is no different. You are all alone, by yourself. No nurse at your side. No patient to tell you the nature of the problem. No office staff. Nobody but yourself. That may be the biggest adjustment for most physicians, because medicine is just the opposite. You can't practice medicine in a closed room all by yourself. There must be someone else in that room. Writing is done in that closed room. Writing is not only solitary, it is lonely. It may not be a good job for a "people person." Discouraged yet? Well, there is another option. If you want to write and yet need people all around you, try writing plays. Find yourself an active theater community, or better yet a playwriting group, and you can give that a shot, Rob. These days, playwriting is a group activity with staged readings and input from actors, actresses, directors, other would-be playwrights. There are so many people there willing and anxious to help you write your play that no one could possibly get lonely. And enough help to drive any other writer into the peace and privacy of that little room. I tried it. More than once, and, believe me, Rob, four walls never looked so good.

And it won't come easy. It won't be automatic. Writing is not like medical education, and learning to write, becoming a writer, is not like taking a residency. Virtually everyone who takes a neurology residency becomes a neurologist—a board certified neurologist with a certificate to prove it. It's the same in obstetrics. And every other field of medicine.

Since I've been here we have had well over seventy neurology residents. Some were brilliant. Some were just average. Some were barely competent, at best. They all completed their residencies. And now they are all specialists. Almost all are board certified. Success. Automatic success. That's what medicine is all about. Everyone has his or her boards. To say nothing of a Medicare provider number. Medicine is a field of success, of acceptance. Of automatic accomplishment. Brace yourself, Rob. It just ain't like that in the real world. I have written over four hundred scientific papers. All of them have been published. They have all found homes. I have no drawer filled with unpublished medical articles. An unpublished medical paper is a nonexistent commodity. Write it, and it will find a home. Perhaps not the *New England Journal of Medicine*, but somewhere.

Writing, especially the writing of fiction, is just the opposite. It is a field of rejection. I'm considered fairly successful as an author. My first novel, *Sins of Omission*, was a Book-of-the-Month Club alternate selection. Think of it, Rob. The Book-of-the-Month Club. On my first try. That's like pitching a no-hitter in your first start in the majors. Could Cooperstown be far away? Success. Triumph! The big time. My first novel. What could be better? Another of my books, *Toscanini's Miscue*, was a Literary Guild alternate selection. My books have been translated into a dozen different languages. Now that's success for you. I have written seven novels. Only three have been published in the United States. The other four have been rejected by twenty or more publishers each. And my second novel, *Jerusalem Plot*, was rejected twenty-three times before it was accepted. So much for my no-hitter. I should have remembered the curse of Bobo Holloman. He pitched a no-hitter in his first major league start for the lowly St. Louis Browns. Before the season was half over, he was back in the minors. No ticket to Cooperstown for him.

Consider what you are giving up. No medical article of mine was ever rejected more than five or six times; no matter how bad it was. And I'll admit it, some of them were not *that* great. And no matter how little they added to our scientific knowledge in the long run, someone published them.

And I'm told that three out of seven is not that bad in this business. Not that bad at all. In fact, that's really pretty damn good. That's a batting average of .429. Not even Ty Cobb hit that high. Nor Rogers Hornsby, who had the highest single season average ever. But I'm not an outfielder. Or a second baseman. I'm a writer. A serious writer. And what's even more frustrating is that I'm a writer who has become accustomed to batting 1.000. Hell, nobody even fields that well. And no one hits that well. So, unless you have a very high level of tolerance for rejection, unless you're willing to subject yourself to that rejection, stick to medicine. Rejection slips are worse than any insurance company's refusal to pay a bill. Much more personal. Much harder to take. They're not merely business as usual; they're a rejection of you. Not the procedure, but you, personally. They always hurt.

By the way, both drafts of this letter, start to finish, took less than the first half of a pro football game. But I took no time-outs. Just lots of replays. Good luck, Rob.

Your friend,

Roger

July 1—11 A.M.

Dear Rob,

I forgot to mention the other subject you brought up in your letter. That shows you where my priorities are these days. Obviously, I am very proud of the article that you read in the *New England Journal of Medicine*. All of us who are part of the Parkinson Study Group are, with various levels of grandiosity and self-indulgence. Taken at face value, if it can be, and all good members of the PSG certainly believe that our research can be taken in that manner and have been so assured by our biostatisticians that it can be, and we of course believe them, then for the first time ever we've shown that the progression of a "degenerative" disease, for that is what Parkinson's disease is classified as—a progressive, degenerative disease—well, that progression of such a disorder can be slowed down. How's that for a complex sentence? That's what happens when you think about science too much. Or read Victor Hugo.

Think about it, Rob. Everything that we do for Parkinson's disease, and we do a lot, but it's all only symptomatic therapy. We replace the missing chemical and treat the symptoms, but the disease goes on. The nerve cells keep right on dying. Well, not any more. We can slow that process down. Slow down the progression of a degenerative disease. Delay the inevitable.

What a breakthrough! We've never been able to do that before for any neurologic disease. But now we can for Parkinson's disease. If we can do it for Parkinson's disease, why not for other degenerative diseases? Why not Alzheimer's? ALS? Why not? Not cure them. Not reverse them. But slow their progression. Stay their course. There is no reason why not. A lifetime of mild Parkinson's disease wouldn't be all bad. Would Lou Gehrig have settled for a lifetime of mild ALS? You bet he would.

It took five years of hard work, a twelve million dollar federal grant, and a lot of luck. But it was worth it. Mylan Pharmaceutical makes the drug. It's called Eldepryl here. Will they make money on it? Hell, yes! That's why they are in the business of developing drugs.

Can you still get in on it and make money on the stock? Ask your broker. Or investment counselor. Or asset manager. Or whomever. But not me. That is not something I do well.

Roger

July 8

Dear Rob:

I'm being sued. Not in a malpractice suit. That I could accept. Malpractice suits have become a normal part of the practice of medicine, part of the overhead. Like rent and payroll taxes. A way of life. Ain't that a fine state of affairs? Well, this is far worse than malpractice. I'm being sued for libel and by someone I've known almost my entire life, even though we've never met.

Who? The famous Martin Bloom. The official caption of the case is *Bloom vs. Kramer et al.* And who, you ask, is this Martin Bloom? A very good question, my friend. He was a pitcher for the White Sox of my youth. The boys of my summer. And, all in all, he was not a very good pitcher. His entire major league career consisted of about forty-five games in which he pitched no more than eighty-five innings. That means he faced a grand total of three hundred and ninety batters, give or take a few hit batters. Altogether that would not even make much of a season. And, let me remind you, it's not one season I'm writing about here

10

but his whole damn career. But it wasn't his pitching ability that had made him one of my heroes. Even at age twelve I was smart enough to recognize that. After all, my White Sox had good pitchers, a lot of them. In '49 we had four of the best young left-handers in all of baseball. Pierce, Kuzava, Wight, Cain. Marty, we always called him Marty back then, Marvelous Marty, was also left-handed, but the resemblance to the other four pretty much ended there. But I didn't care, he was a hero of mine. Why? Because he was Jewish, one of a few Jews playing for my Chicago White Sox. There was another lefty named Rotblatt and one who was really important, a right-handed pitcher named Rogovin. Somnolent Saul Rogovin. We got him in a trade from Detroit for one of our left-handers, Bob Cain. Rogovin became a star as we battled for the pennant. He won a dozen games in 1951. He also had the best earned run average in the league. I was going to write ERA, but that acronym has gained a new meaning over the years.

Bob Cain, by the way, the left-hander we traded to get Saul Rogovin, went on to another form of glory, more important than leading the league in ERA. He was the pitcher for Detroit when Bill Veeck, then the owner of the hapless St. Louis Browns, used a midget as a pinch hitter. Eddie Gaedel. He wore number one-half and was used once as a pinch hitter, and Bob Cain pitched to Eddie Gaedel. Cain walked him on four pitches. Laughing all the time. The league made Veeck fire Gaedel. I don't think they could do that today. I mean Veeck had to fire Gaedel because he was a midget, he had to fire him because of a medical condition. Gaedel was an achondroplastic dwarf. That has to be unconstitutional. Midgets of the world, arise! You can do more than be in the chorus in *The Wizard of Oz*.

Back to Marvelous Marty. So he sued me. Why?

Because I used his name.

Did I use it intentionally? Hell, yes. Of that I am guilty. Guilty as charged. But of what? Why did I do it? Why? The answer is obvious. As obvious as a Martin Bloom fast ball on a 3 and 1 count. I did it as a tribute to him as one of my childhood heroes. And the SOB sued me. So much for sports heroes.

I guess I ought to go back to the beginning. No, not to '51, just back to '75. I was writing my first novel back then and I had one apparently insurmountable problem that was driving me crazy. Not the intricate plot. Not maintaining the suspense. Not devising a new and previously unused means of carrying out a murder. That was mere child's play. As a neurologist interested in pharmacology and toxicology, I had dozens to choose from. I'm sure you, as a gynecologist, could devise some real lulus. How about a tampon soaked with penicillin self-inserted by a patient with a past history of severe anaphylactic shock from penicillin? She puts in the tampon before going to bed and wakes up dead. Who would ever check her tampon for penicillin? Sperm? Perhaps. Blood. But penicillin? A perfect crime. But I digress. What was my problem? Names. I am, as I have said before, terrible with names. I can't remember them. I can't keep them straight. And here I had a book with nothing but names. Names galore, as Ian Fleming would have put it. Doctors, patients, residents, medical students. Hell, eight people get killed in the first seven chapters. How could I remember who got killed, which patient was which, which medical student?

Easy. I'd give them names I already knew and I'd give them names with built-in associations that would help me keep them all in order.

What names? That was obvious. Old ballplayers.

Which ones? Mostly old White Sox, of course.

My hero, the neurologist and head of the Department of Neurology, took the name of the White Sox manager who led us out of the doldrums of second division into pennant contention, Paul Richards. The other neurologists became his coaches. Lum Harris, Don Gutteridge. Simple. Easy. Helpful. And fun. That's what I was writing the novel for, fun. Not for publication, but to see if I could actually write a novel. So what about the eight murder victims? New York Yankees. Who else did I want to kill? Too obvious. All of their names were far too well known. Everybody knows Mickey Mantle and Yogi Berra. To say nothing of Jolting Joe. I settled on the starting lineup of the Cleveland Indians, not in order, however. The first victim was not leadoff man, Dale Mitchell, but cleanup hitter, Al Rosen. Not as Al Rosen, but as the wife of Rabbi Rosen.

My best was naming one of the residents Herb Adams, part-time center fielder for the White Sox in 1950, and naming his girlfriend Gerri Scala. The real Jerry Scala was the guy who alternated in center field with Herb Adams in Comiskey Park in 1950. So they shared a bed in my book. Good clean fun. And nobody got hurt. Or libeled in any way.

Then in 1981 I sent the book to Burt Shapiro. He is what is meant by *et al*. Burt, then and now, is president and owner of Sharp Books, which is said, by Burt, to be the largest trade publisher outside of New York City. It certainly is one of the largest in the Midwest. So after my book had languished in a drawer in an all but discarded desk in the basement for six years, I finally submitted my fun novel to a publisher and, to my dismay, Burt accepted it and, as the saying goes, the rest is history.

During the editorial process, while we were at lunch one day at his club on the sixty-fifth floor of the Standard Oil Building overlooking Lake Michigan, we were discussing our book. I liked his having such a proprietary interest. "Our" book. I mentioned the name game to Burt. By the way, none of my subsequent New York publishers has ever taken me to lunch. One editor did give me a cup of coffee once. In a styrofoam cup. In a room without a window, much less a view.

"You can't do that," he bellowed.

"Why?"

"They could sue you." Emphasis on the "you." His emphasis, not mine.

"Me?" I asked.

"It's your book," he informed me.

Whatever had happened to "our" book, I wondered.

"You," he repeated for emphasis.

"For what?"

"Defamation of character!"

"Defamation. How could you defame someone who never managed to hit .200? Like Jerry Scala? Or Marty Bloom? He was not exactly a three hundred game winner. He only won five games in his entire lifetime. Even among Jewish pitchers, that's about as low as you can get. Even among Jewish White Sox pitchers. Barry Latman won more than that in '59. Hell, you can't defame guys like that." I carefully made no mention of Hall of Fame third baseman Al Rosen. In my book he'd undergone a sex change operation of sorts. Nor did I mention any of the other good players.

"Invasion of privacy," he countered tenaciously. Maybe it's a good thing that I haven't gone to lunch with any other publisher.

"I'm not invading their privacy. I'm not writing about a guy named Marty Bloom who pitched for the White Sox. I'm writing about a patient with a bad disease who happened to have the same name."

"Change the names."

"Suppose I'd named my character Al Smith after our left fielder in '59?"

"Change them."

"Could the Democratic candidate for President in '28 sue me?"

"Change them."

It was an order. I had to change them. How? To what? Gloom. Doom. The prospect of coming up with all those names all over again appalled me. It depressed me. It aggravated me. I wanted to pay homage to some of those old White Sox players.

13

Change them! To what? To whom? Then I figured out a solution. Instead of the names of old ballplayers I used the names of old physicians, dead physicians, physicians who had described obscure diseases. Physicians whose names I now knew as well as I knew those of old ballplayers. That became my game. Lum Harris became two pathologists: Arnold and Chiari. Together they had described one of the major congenital abnormalities of the brain—the Arnold-Chiari malformation. But Chiari also described thrombosis of the veins of the liver. He did that along with another pathologist named Budd—the Budd-Chiari syndrome. So Arnold Chiari acquired a nickname—"Bud."

It was a new game. Herb Adams became Herb Westfall. And Gerri Scala became Gerri Edinger. Why Westfall? Why Edinger? Because together those two men described one nucleus in the brain, the Edinger-Westfall nucleus. Sharing a nucleus is not too far removed from sharing a bed. At least as close as playing in the same outfield.

And what happened to Paul Richards? I liked that name, so I just made a minor change. He became Paul Richardson. But in so doing, his wife was transformed from Bobbie Richards *sui generis* to Bobbie Richardson, all-star second baseman for the hated New York Yankees. No wonder I killed her off between my first novel and my second novel. A fatal spot. Wouldn't you have done the same thing? Playing for the New York Yankees. The traitor! As bad as David Garron refusing to take treatment for his gout. Benedict Arnold had nothing on either of them. She deserved being killed.

But I didn't change everything. In one section of the book, Paul Richardson, né Richards, as part of a research project, reviews a number of hospital charts, random names followed by six-digit hospital numbers.

Random, hell. Those names come directly from the lineup of the '48 Boston Braves and the six-digit hospital number was each player's own numbers—his batting average plus his slugging percentage, or fielding average, or win-loss percentage, or earned run average. An example: A. Dark. Alvin Dark. All-star shortstop. He hit .322 that year and had a slugging percentage of .433. So the entry became A. Dark, #322-433.

Another example: I'll take a pitcher this time. They use different statistics. V. Bickford. Vern Bickford. Their third starting pitcher. They had three. It was not just Spahn, Sain, and pray for rain. Bickford had a win-loss percentage of .688 and an earned run average of .327. V. Bickford, #688-327.

And I made an intentional error. For one of the players I used the '49 statistics. Which one? I'll never tell. So far six readers have caught this error and taken the time to write to me about it. Several even chastised me for my carelessness. By the way, without looking at the book, I can't tell you what name I gave to the patient I had originally christened Marty Bloom, but it sure as hell wasn't Marty Bloom. You can bet on that.

So much for background. On to my "libelous" tort. Or should I say my supposedly libelous tort? Or my supposed libelous alleged tort?

My first nonfiction book was also published by Sharp Books six years after my novel. The return of Burt Shapiro. And more lunches in his club overlooking Lake Michigan. Much nicer than coffee out of a styrofoam cup in a windowless cubicle in New York City, where I had a big-time, big-city publisher and I'd really had it made. The book was called *Toscanini's Miscue*, and it was a set of clinical tales. One of them was about the same patient I had not called Marty Bloom in *Sins of Omission*. This time I called him Marty Bloom. It wasn't about *the* Marty Bloom. That was clear in the story. The Marty Bloom in my story went into his dad's business selling real estate and never played baseball. So much for facts. But I also made it quite clear that this was not the patient's real name. I wrote that I had written about the patient I have "called Marty Bloom" once before . . . in *Sins of Omission*.

In another chapter of the same book, I wrote about a ballplayer who was my patient and told the reader all about my use of old ballplayers' names in the first draft of my first novel. I related how I didn't use the names of stars like Minnie Minoso or Nellie Fox, but those poorly recalled, less-than-journeymen players whom only we few die-hard nuts still remembered—the Al Kozars and Gordon Goldsberrys of this world. Thus Al Kozar had become my patient, transformed magically into Allison Kozar. And the next chapter introduced a patient named . . . Allison Kozar. You didn't have to be a genius to figure out what I was doing. Even the senior editor at Sharp Books figured it out. He called me to discuss my "problem." I discussed *the* problem with him. He decided to publish the book without changing the names.

The book came out that way and Marty has sued me. He sued me *et al*. Me and Sharp Books. Why? Because his best friend read the book and thought that Marty was dead. And had been for years. Some best friend. I wonder if David thinks I'm dead.

I hope Marty doesn't tell Al Kozar what I did. Or Bobbie Richardson. They've become women in my book. God knows what they could sue me for. And Luke Appling. The most famous White Sox player of them all. I never even used his name. That must be the worst insult of all. But he can't sue me. He's dead. R.I.P.

Perhaps this too is part of the curse of Bobo Holloman. Hubris revisited.

See you in court,

Roger

July 11

Dear Rob,

I just reread my first letter to you and there a few things I skipped. I know the advice that others must have already given you. It's simple. If you want to learn how to write, start writing. My advice to people who want to write is to start reading. I have given this same advice to every medical student and every resident who was about to start his or her first paper: read. And now I'm giving it to you. Read, but read to learn, not to be entertained. Read Hemingway. Read Steinbeck. Read Cheever. Read Vonnegut. Updike. Even Conan Doyle. Real writers. But read them as if they were textbooks, medical textbooks. Underline them. Highlight them. All the good descriptions. The sentences that pack a wallop. The thoughts that are well conveyed. Then go back and study them. The same way you studied anatomy. Neuroanatomy. Gynecology. Figure out why those authors worked for you. Why those descriptions hit you. Those thoughts. Those phrases. Those paragraphs. Those chapters. Those books. Rewrite those descriptions you love. Apply them to what you want to write. Plagiarize! Steal from the best. Call it research. Just don't publish it.

How do you know who to read? As an author, you will start to read very differently. I used to read voraciously and finished every book I ever started, even James Joyce. Not *Finnegan's Wake*. I have it on good authority that no one who was not working on a Ph.D. thesis ever finished *Finnegan's Wake*. Today I finish far fewer books. Why? I read for style, for substance, not for plot. Not to be entertained. A poorly written best-seller aggravates me. It is, I hope, more than just jealousy on my part, but jealousy, at least, is an honest emotion. I also read for structure. Mysteries that hide facts and in so doing cheat on the reader are anathema to me. I've thrown them away with forty pages to go, or less. You know just what I mean. The detective finds the clue but doesn't tell you what it is. So all you learn is that the author couldn't maintain suspense except by hiding facts from the reader. Big deal. Any idiot can do that. It's called lying. It's not the denouement that is important. Not the climax. It's the foreplay that counts. Ask your wife. Ask your mistress. Ask your patients. They'll all agree with me.

When my first novel was accepted for publication, I reread it for the first time in five years. I was appalled by its deficiencies in style and structure. Not appalled enough to withdraw it. Never that. I am a writer. But appalled enough to want to rewrite it. The publisher told me that the editorial comments would be done in six weeks, then I could incorporate them into my revisions. What could I do in those six weeks to get ready? I could read. But what?

For style: Hemingway. *A Farewell to Arms*, *The Sun Also Rises*.

For telling a story: Graham Greene's *The Third Man*, Eric Ambler's *A Coffin for Dimitrious*, Conrad's *Heart of Darkness*. The first two also served for pacing.

For direct communication: Vonnegut's *Mother Night*.

And since I was writing a mystery, some of the Conan Doyle canon, including *The Hound of the Baskervilles*. And early Nicholas Freeling.

Construct your own list. Not necessarily of your favorite books. My list contains some of my favorites but not all the ones I chose to read are in my top ten. Those I picked to study were chosen to help me become a better writer with my own style of writing, with my own way of telling the story. There was no place in that list for Kazantzakis. No place for any translations. No Simenon. Nor Gide. Nor Grass. Not even Chekhov. And no place for Faulkner. No place at all. Not my style.

Try it, Rob. As they say, give it your best shot. Make a list of authors whose way of telling a story you like or whose style you admire and reread them. Again and again. With pen in hand, or highlighter. If you cannot construct such a list, what you are aspiring to become may be a medical journalist, not an author. There is a difference.

I can hear you now. What you're thinking is that you don't have to do all that, all you need is a good editor. Getting a good editor is not easy. I've worked with over a dozen. Only a couple of them ever added to what I was doing in any significant way. You have to learn to be your own editor. That is most of what writing is. It's editing. It's rewriting. That college course should have been called creative rewriting. And it's mostly self-criticism. And that's not easy. But you have friends who could help you. If they're not writers, they won't help you. Why not? Two reasons. First, you will quickly realize that, if asked, anyone can be a critic and editor. No skill is needed. No experience. No understanding of your needs. Just the ability to read. Free advice is worth exactly what you pay for it. That's also the second reason. You will not have any faith in their advice. And you shouldn't.

So you must learn your own style. And not to be self-indulgent. That's the hardest part. All of us are, by profession, self-indulgent. You chose obstetrics and gynecology because that was what you wanted to do. Why, I'll never know, but it appealed to you, so that is what you do. All day long. I became a neurologist because that's what I wanted to do. That's medicine. We do surgery because we like to. Or don't because we don't. We do what we want to do when we want to do it, where we want to do it, and get paid very well for it. If this doesn't describe you, it ought to. And to correct it, change your medical life. Learning to write, publishing a book, won't change your professional life.

Cut the self-indulgence. Not every word I write is worth reading. Nor will every word you write. Leave self-indulgence to James Joyce and Ezra Pound. Fewer people have read *The Cantos* than have read *Finnegan's Wake* and justifiably so. But you want to be read. If not that, then why write? If you want to be self-indulgent, take another fellowship, learn a new procedure. Start a sleep lab. Be the first in your neighborhood to test balance. The number of gimmicks in medicine is unlimited. Go for it.

But expression is the need of your soul. Be careful when you say that, Rob; people tend to become what they pretend to be, so don't pretend. But if you still feel the need, then you should try to write. But it's not like collecting art. Or building model planes. If you aren't good at it, you will fail miserably. And if you are, you will still fail to some degree, and despite all that failure, it's addicting; as addicting as any human activity can be. Be warned. Writing may be dangerous to the rest of your life.

Roger

July 15—9 A.M.
Via FAX

Dear Rob,

Write. Do not call. In fact, do not ever call me again. I only took your call because I thought it was about a patient—most doctors still call me about patients, sick patients, patients with whom they need help or advice, real emergencies. Not advice on starting a novel.

Next time I will not respond. If you call, I will not answer. If I answer, I will not talk. Sherman had nothing on me. If I wanted to tell you these things over the phone, I'd call you. But don't sit by the phone waiting; I won't call.

Why not? The spoken word is not the written word. While spontaneity may be lost in a letter, everything else is gained.

And besides, there can never be *The Collected Phone Calls of Roger Kramer.* Letters last. Phone calls end when you hang up. They are for once and then they are nothing. If they ever were.

Roger

July 21

Dear Rob,

Do not, repeat *do not*, open a sleep lab. There are already too many of those run by people who don't really know what they are doing. Mostly physicians who practice pulmonary medicine as far as I can tell. Hopefully, they know something about pulmonary medicine, although I am skeptical. I do know about sleep disorders. Most of them are neurologic disorders. Not pulmonary diseases.

Two months ago I saw a patient from southern Illinois. Somewhere around Cairo. We say "Kay-ro," not Cairo. As if the town were named after the syrup, not the capital of Egypt. The patient was referred to me because he had muscle jerks as he was falling asleep. They were sudden movements, more like spasms. Spasms. So he was sent to me. After all, I am supposed to be an expert on abnormal movements.

Could he remember the movements? No.

19

Could he describe them? No.

Could his wife? Not well.

Was he already asleep when the jerks occurred? He wasn't certain. Nor was she.

Did they involve one leg or both? Yes. Or no. Neither of them was certain. Neither was exactly a Toynbee. So many patients don't realize that's their job. They have to be the historians of their health.

Did the jerks involve both the arm and leg? They were both asleep.

Was the movement a single jerk? Or a succession of similar movements? Another unanswered question.

Fast or slow? . . . But why go on?

"You need a sleep study," I said.

"What's that?" they asked.

I explained. He'd come into our sleep lab and be hooked up to an EEG machine that would record the activity of his brain, and we'd also record his eye movements and breathing patterns and muscle activity, all at the same time, and he would also be videotaped. That way we could review everything at once, breathing, brain waves, muscle tone, and also the movements. Then we would know what the movements looked like, where they came from, what caused them, and how to treat them. There were answers we could only obtain by simultaneously seeing what we had to see on the EEG and videotape. Such as: Is he really asleep when the jerks appear? The EEG would show that. In what stage of sleep do the jerks occur? That we'd see by comparing the EEG and the muscle tone and the eye movements and the videotape. What do the movements look like? We'd see that on the videotape. Were they single or in flurries? Were they sudden, rapid jerks or slower movements? Did they involve one leg or both? Was the arm involved? Did the EEG change when the movements occurred? If so, what did the EEG discharge look like? That would tell us if these were seizures or not, and what kinds of medicines to try.

Sounded good to him. And his wife.

He came back today. Report in hand. He didn't have his sleep study here. Why? His HMO only approves local tests whenever available.

The report was a thing of beauty:

Complaint: Jerks on going to sleep.

Observation: Jerks on going to sleep.

Conclusion: Jerks on going to sleep.

Signed: Some jerk who is a pulmonologist who runs a sleep lab.

Was the patient asleep when the jerks occurred? The pulmonologist never said one way or the other. What stage of sleep was the patient in?

Not noted. What did the jerks look like? No mention, not by our friend the pulmonologist. Was one leg involved or both? Did the movements occur as single events or in flurries? Did the EEG change? The EEG? That was never mentioned.

Do you know why Jesus was put in a manger when He was born? Because Joseph belonged to an HMO.

A medical joke. As far as I could tell, Joseph's HMO also had a contract with this pulmonologist to do sleep studies. He is far cheaper than our lab. But we sometimes know what we're doing.

So, Rob, please do not open a sleep lab. I'm sure it would be a moneymaker for your practice. But does your practice really need the money? Or is that question tantamount to heresy? Don't get into sleep. I have enough trouble with the labs that are already operating without any concept of what they're doing.

On a happier note, I wanted to tell you that my batting average is about to change, irrevocably, for the better or the worse. That's right, I've finished another novel. It's another hospital-based mystery with my favorite neurologist-turned-sleuth, Paul Richardson. I just sent it off to my agent and in a couple of days, long enough so that I'll know he's had time to read it, but not long enough to have read it carefully and critiqued it, or even have given it a modicum of editorial commentary, he will call me and tell me that it is brilliant, my best yet, a sure sell, more taut than anything I've done before, more suspenseful, worthy of a far larger advance, six figures at least. Certainly a ripe candidate for a combined hardcover/paperback deal. The novel itself is about AIDS. My tentative title is *The Blind Observer* and while it does involve good ol' Paul Richardson, the main character for the first two-thirds is a young woman who has a Master of Public Health from Johns Hopkins and who now works at Austin Flint Medical Center as a biostatistician and epidemiologist. She gets involved in tracing the source of HIV infection in an AIDS patient who is murdered in the hospital. The source was a blood transfusion the patient received in 1982. Arthur Ashe revisited!

But was that the source? And, if so, which donor has AIDS? The search for the HIV-positive donor. Or all you ever wanted to know about AIDS but were afraid to ask. How safe is the blood supply? How safe is safe sex? Homosexual? Heterosexual? Oral? Vaginal? Anal? What have you? To do her job, she must answer these and other questions. All within the fabric of a complex mystery. An easy sell? I doubt it. Who wants to read a novel about AIDS? Not the P.D. James and Agatha Christie fans, that's for damn sure!

But it's done. Off to my agent. My denominator is now up. From seven to eight. In a few months we'll know about the numerator. Four for eight is .500. Three for eight is .375. Ty Cobb's lifetime batting average, the highest in the history of the game, was only .367. I am not, I remind you, a right fielder. I did not go to medical school to learn how to hit a curve ball. The sad fact is that I never learned to hit a curve ball. A great tragedy to which I am still adjusting. Me and Frank Miller. He was first cellist for the Chicago Symphony. Also for Toscanini. The greatest orchestral cellist of this century. He became a cellist when he realized he couldn't hit a curve.

Roger

July 23

Dear Rob:

David Garron came by my office today. David is my best friend at the medical school. He has been for many, many years. He would be a best friend even without our professional relationship. When we're both in town, he averages almost two visits per week. David claims he remembers me from my internship. I do not doubt him, but I do not remember him from then, so I'm sure you don't. Our relationship goes back almost twenty-five years. We were brought together to answer a research question about the side effects of levodopa. We worked together to design a protocol and to carry it out. It was a good study. Nothing revolutionary. Nothing startling. It was published, of course. And is still mentioned in the literature from time to time. We made no great discoveries. Except that he knew Beckett and Gide and Auden and Kazantzakis. And so did I. David is a neuropsychologist and is, in many ways, a fish out of water. He was trained as a Freudian psychologist but he practices as a neuropsychologist doing various psychologic tests on patients with neurologic disorders to tease out which problems may be neurologic in origin and which may not.

And he never treats anyone. He is a true consultant. What I originally thought I wanted to be. One visit and he is through. But it is never slam, bam, thank you ma'am. Never. Not with David. His visits take forever. And not just the testing. He is a true student of narrative. Each person is a story and David always takes the time to ferret out that story. Piece by piece. Year by year. Nuance by nuance. The story, he says, helps him choose which tests to run. And his diagnosis is, he maintains, always based on the test results. It is the narrative that allows him to exercise his clinical acumen. That he readily admits. And his acumen is unexcelled as far as I'm concerned. I'm never sure it really comes from the testing and not from the story itself, but perhaps that's my prejudice. My diagnosis almost always comes from the story. Not the examination, the story.

David is not an M.D. Not a physician. So in a way he must always be an outsider. I, too, am an outsider here, but for me that is more by choice. I observe my fellow physicians far more than I share their lives. I always have. Who else carried a copy of Gide in his pocket during his internship? Or Camus? Or Beckett? Not the Wash Manual, or some other medical text. All you ever needed to know in six hundred crowded pages. Even Joyce would have been better company than that. But not Pound. Never Pound.

Perhaps what David remembers is that copy of Rilke that was in my pocket during my internship.

So David comes by and we talk of many things. Often he tells me a story. One he obtained from one of his patients. Occasionally one from a patient of mine. We rarely talk about research during these impromptu get-togethers, although we've done collaborative research ever since '68. Research on Parkinson's disease. Research on Huntington's disease. Problems in these diseases where neurology and neuropsychology overlap. Those problems are still there so we sometimes dissect a new research idea, an approach to a problem, but not the design of a study. Mostly we talk about literature. Literary characters. Writers. Their lives as much as their works. Their narratives. The people who peopled their lives. Such rich diversity. Alma Mahler. Osip Mandelstam. Siegfried Sassoon. Especially Sassoon. David has a major interest in Sassoon. Sassoon was the first great poet of the trenches in World War I, the Great War. He made a poet of Wilfred Owen. He was the first literary figure to turn against the war. He then spent much of his life after that war creating his own persona. It's that which fascinates David. Like Oscar Wilde creating Oscar Wilde. Only Sassoon, the Baghdad Jew, became the ultimate Englishman. Someday David hopes to write a book on Sassoon. David is also a writer. He writes short stories. I have never read a single one. He has not shown me one. I've never asked to see one. Why not? And why not? I cannot tell you why he has not shown me any. That's been his decision. I've never asked because our friendship has always been made up of the analysis of whatever each of us brings into the conversation. No outward probing. No questions about my divorce. Only the frank discussion of issues I brought up. No holds barred, but on my terms. With the limits I set. So I have never asked. I wait. I will read them some day.

David also wants to be a full-time writer. When he retires. No affairs for David. He may lust in his heart, and he does, but not with his body. One love at a time.

Today he hobbled into my office, and I do mean hobbled. With a capital H. He has gout. Classic gout with the sudden onset of severe pain in the great toe. The first joint of the great toe. His left great toe. Ben Franklin revisited. He could not even wear a shoe. Or talk of Sassoon.

When had it started? A week ago. No wonder I hadn't seen him for over a week. "What are you on?" I asked.

"Nothing."

For the briefest of instances, I was dumbfounded. Even Ben Franklin had taken something. Colchicine. A tea made from bark of the cinchona tree. Franklin had helped to introduce that to America as a treatment for gout. But in a moment I recovered. And once I had reconsidered the character and the situation, I was no longer even surprised. It was pure David. David, the student of the natural history of disease. Even as I asked him why he was on no medication, I knew pretty much what he would say.

Gout always goes away. It always has. A first attack is never a permanent condition. True, it is a harbinger of a permanent, inherited metabolic disorder. But the acute attack always goes away. Ben Franklin's did. David Garron knew that his would.

"Franklin took colchicine," I reminded him.

"Not for his first attack."

"Touché."

"And that's a terrible drug. Nausea, diarrhea, ..."

"I know. I'm a pharmacologist, remember?"

He ignored my self-aggrandizement. He always does. He's sixty. Gout at sixty virtually always goes away within four to six weeks and usually does not come back. So he was on nothing.

No medication at all?

None.

I wished him good luck.

He had a high pain threshold, he reminded me. But pain, I told him, would not be his problem. I don't think he understood. But that is because he is not one of us. He has rejected one of the tenets of modern medicine. The rest of his friends, the ones who supply most of his consultations, the ones who would think that Siegfried Sassoon is Vidal's father, they will not understand his decision. They are doctors, treating physicians. They believe their own myths. And he has figuratively slapped each of them in the face. After they had allowed him into their club. So I wished him luck. He'll need it.

Roger

Sunday, July 28, 5:30 A.M.

Dear Rob,

I've been reading again. I do mean again. I read in spurts. I've been reading Rilke. I think it was my mention of him in my last letter to you that got me started. I probably haven't read anything of his in twenty years. I've been making up for lost time. I started with *The Notebooks of Malte Laurids Brigge* and then went on to his letters. I am getting into reading letters. Following my own advice. Like all good writers, Rilke has made me think about both his writings and mine. I am certainly no Rainer Maria Rilke. Nor do I pretend to be. Nor aspire to be. Don't get me wrong; that does not mean that I do not have lofty literary aspirations. Because I certainly do. Aspirations that may be far above any reasonable expectations on my part and equally far beyond my control. But what's wrong with expectations? Just call them dreams or fantasies and they become quite acceptable. I recognize, as Rilke did, that I have a divided allegiance.

That was what bothered you most. And what Chekhov lied about. But who doesn't? There must always be some conflict between the needs of your art, the dedication that it demands, the time, the concentration, the energy, the libidinal commitment, and the needs of the rest of your life. This conflict may seem far greater if you're a doctor, but that does not make it any different, and even if it did, this issue would not become some primal existentialist conflict. It is not some rarified conundrum reserved only for creative geniuses. Rilke got that all wrong. It was the arrogant romantic in him. He knew he was a great artist. He was struggling. Ergo, great artists struggle. Ergo, heroic struggling is the purview of great artists.

I've got news for him, bad artists struggle. So do most people. It is the stuff of both everyday life and art. It is what life and literature are all about. It is part of the human condition, not an existential philosophical debate. It is the same struggle we all go through, defining ourselves independent of our work. I am not just a doctor. My secretary does not exist solely to be a secretary. Rilke's struggle was not qualitatively different. Quantitatively perhaps. But not qualitatively. That is a truth I accept.

Was Cézanne the man who resolved that conflict most completely? Rilke thought that Cézanne was the epitome of dedication to his creative art. Cézanne had became one with his art. So much that he missed his mother's funeral. And did that make Cézanne the purest of the pure? The artist par excellence? The one of many? The pure, dedicated artist? Or was he no different from the rest of us? A man who had resolved his own crisis in the way that was best for him as an artist. And as a struggling individual beset by nonartistic problems and conflicts. Like his grocer, and his wine merchant, and the guys he watched playing cards during those evenings before TV. He was a struggling personality, not a model to be emulated. And we applaud Cézanne because by solving his crisis we, the rest of mankind, reaped the profits—those wonderful, nonspontaneous surfaces peopled primarily not by people. Apples much more than people. So we are all to applaud, to cheer, to understand Cézanne's decision to stay away from his mother's funeral in order not to miss a day of painting. He did that for his art and for us, for posterity. For crying out loud! I don't understand why he did that. And I certainly don't empathize. And I neither thank him nor applaud him. Missing his mother's funeral was wrong. It was an unforgivable wrong. An inhuman act. What he did was not dedication. Nor should it ever be interpreted as such. It was acting out. Freud would have recognized it as such and so must the rest of us, artists and nonartists alike. It was the action of an angry, spiteful, arrogant little boy. Not that of a responsible adult. And what a degree of arrogance. Better he should have gone. The world would have survived quite well with one less apple. No matter how perfect that apple.

Rilke looked at works of Cézanne and suddenly understood that his life had to belong to his own creations, to his poetry. Before Rilke stood in front of one of those innumerable oils of Mont Sainte Victoire, not quite as ubiquitous as apples, but more so than nudes, and infinitely more than children at play, before that moment, that flash of insight, what had Rilke been doing? Playing at poetry? Pretending to be a poet?

So that became Rilke's crisis. He knew what he had to do. That was

26

his resolution, his commitment. He would follow in Cézanne's footsteps
and like Cézanne become a prophet, a saint. And only experience
delight and awe through his art.

And miss his mother's funeral! And his father's! And his wife's? No
prophet would have done that. No biblical figure who behaved in that way
could have been one of God's prophets. For that transgresses everything
that God is about. It is forbidden to them by God's laws. By their own sense
of human decencies, by their own spiritual needs. Honor thy father and thy
mother. Go to the funeral, buddy. That's what life is all about.

Must you be dedicated to your art? Absolutely. If it's only a game you
want to play, play the games others play. Drive race cars. Take up skiing.
Dabble in real estate. Play the stock market.

But don't believe that you have to give up life. It's not true. Cézanne
did not have to. Picasso never did. Although he never did paint very
many apples. And he made even greater strides than Cézanne in differ-
entiating the reality of the world and the reality of a painting, of reversing the flow of art history. A canvas is not the world. A canvas is flat. It
can never be other than flat. Use that flatness, that surface, don't try to
apologize for it. Don't disguise it. That's what twentieth century art is all
about. Thanks more to Picasso than to Cézanne. And to Braque. And to
Matisse. Flatness and color. There is only one God, but Cézanne was not
His prophet.

So I do not aspire to follow in Rilke's footsteps, in Cézanne's, in the
footsteps of the prophets! Hell, no.

I have two aspirations. They are so different, yet they are also insepa-
rable. I want to be taken seriously as an artist, as a writer. That's both of
them. Create a serious body of work and be taken seriously. One I strive
for, the other is beyond my control.

In medicine we are all taken so damn seriously. Perhaps too seriously. It comes with the territory. I am no Louis Pasteur. I never will
be. I never wanted to be. I never had any aspirations of Nobel Prize
proportions. I know people who do. Or at one time did. I've worked
with them. Coauthored papers together. I know people who have
won Nobel Prizes. I'm not in that league. Never was. Never will be.
Never dreamed I would be. In medicine I just wanted to do what I
wanted to do, to do it well and be taken seriously. What did I want to
do? That's not an easy question to answer. I wanted to see if it really
made sense. Did the facts the real scientists were learning, those who
won Nobel Prizes, like Axelrod and von Eulenberg, and those who
should have, like Arvid Carlson, could their facts be applied at the

bedside and be converted into better lives for my patients? *And* could I translate what happened to my patients into scientific facts? And be taken seriously?

I did all of that and I am taken seriously, all too seriously sometimes. There are instances when an experiment is only that. At times it is only an exercise in collecting data. Like a cigar can at times be nothing more than a good smoke, a good smoke that is a risk factor for cancer of the throat. Not every piece of data is worth analyzing. And not every analysis is worth interpreting. And not every interpretation is worth publishing.

Collecting data is like writing sentences. A writer writes them all the time. And sometimes puts them together in a meaningful way and publishes them. If only science were like that. Data collection is not progress. It is not an end in and of itself. The Great American Experiment. And no one should pretend that it is.

Being taken seriously in medicine wasn't all that easy. I did clinical research. I studied patients. Not rats, marmosets, or even guinea pigs. People. Better it should have been apples. People are not pure science. The results are not clear enough. They neither abstract not controllable. That made my work too unreliable, too unclean. Far too unclean. It wasn't real science.

What a crock!

What is medical science all about? It has to be about the application of real data to real patients. The observation that a procedure cures experimental parkinsonism in a monkey is all well and good—if your desire is to treat monkeys, monkeys whose parkinsonism you caused. But I take care of sick people.

Clinical research is the mystery genre of medical science. A mystery may be a novel but it isn't literature. Hammett never won a National Book Award. He may have helped Lillian Hellman win a Pulitzer Prize but you really couldn't take that story about that blackbird seriously. So what if in a single sentence he changed the direction of the entire genre. You must know which one I mean. His partner has been killed and the cops have called Sam Spade to come to the scene. Spade and one of the cops are looking over a precipice at the body. The cop asks Spade if he wants to look at the body. He doesn't. He tells the cop that he couldn't see anything that they hadn't already seen. TILT. Prior to that, the detective hero was modeled on Sherlock Holmes and possessed superior powers of observation. Or on Hercule Poirot with his magnificent little grey cells. Not any more. Sam Spade threw down the gauntlet and the field was changed forever. To the world of literature, that was no more significant than a new batting technique. And his style is also not to be taken seriously. More like the sports pages than literature. As bad as Ring Lardner.

And neither was clinical research to be taken seriously as a discipline. It was a necessary evil. But that may be changing. Not because science is changing. Never. Just the opposite. But people are demanding results. Not facts. Applications. And those of us who do clinical research are no longer shy about what we do. We no longer hide in the closet waiting for the last hour on the last afternoon of a meeting to sneak in our presentations. If it's a meeting about Parkinson's disease, let's talk about patients. Unclean!

There is now a Hammett Award. Given by the International Association of Crime Writers. Not a Pulitzer Prize, true, but it's a start.

Roger

July 28

.

Dear Rob,

Who was Rilke? Do I have to ask if you know who Cézanne was? Sorry. Look him up. Rilke, I mean, not Cézanne. He's even in your kid's *World Book Encyclopedia*. In between James Whitcomb Riley, another poet who was Rilke's contemporary and who is not yet forgotten sufficiently, and Arthur Rimbaud, the French poet who is better remembered than Riley. There may be some poetic justice in this world. Rilke was one of the most important German poets of the first part of this century. A very important poet. The most important German poet between Heine and Brecht. Look them up, too. You might even read something by one of them. Try Brecht first. He wrote *The Threepenny Opera* and *Mother Courage*. Start with the latter. The former only works with the music, which Brecht didn't write.

I'd like you to check out a story for me, if you can do it without going to too much trouble. I've been told by an invariably reliable source about an article that appeared in the *L.A. Times* quite recently, meaning sometime in the last week or two. I'm sure it must have been this month. The story was about a neurosurgeon in Mexico City who is doing adrenal implants in patients with Parkinson's disease and apparently having spectacular results. Good enough to sell newspapers. The results have already stirred up the hopes of more than a fair number of Parkinson patients all over the world.

I'm not exaggerating. That's how I heard about the story. I got a phone call from Geneva. Switzerland, not Wisconsin. Since it was a call from a patient of mine with Parkinson's disease, I did talk to him. Referring to him as my patient is only partially accurate. I've seen him only once and that was about eight years ago and that was only to confirm the diagnosis. I have never been his actual treating physician. He's been treated by neurologists in Paris and London, with an occasional stop in Zurich and New York. I guess if I could pick places to go for treatment of my Parkinson's disease, I'd choose London and Paris over Chicago. But I'm not sure that location is the critical factor.

There is no question but that he has PD. There was no question about it when I first saw him over eight years ago. After all these years PD remains just what it was when we were interns together. It is still a clinical diagnosis. There are still no tests for PD. PD, like beauty, is in the eye of the beholder.

Do you remember how to diagnose PD? I doubt it. Why should you? Do I remember how to diagnose a tubal pregnancy? Or even how to do a pelvic examination? Don't ask. Pelvic exams were one of the main reasons I went into neurology. I'd never have to do another pelvic examination. Nor ever pass another proctoscope.

So I will remind you what PD is. No, you don't have to remind me how to pass a vaginal speculum. It is a skill I'm all too happy to have lost completely. PD has four different types of symptoms: tremor, rigidity, bradykinesia, and imbalance. The tremor is called a resting tremor. It is a rhythmic abnormal movement of the hands and fingers that is more marked at rest than during activity. The first time I saw him, my patient from Geneva, his name is Gould, by the way, Fred Gould, I didn't even have to take him into the exam room to see his tremor. It was there whenever either hand was at rest. So I already knew he had one out of the four components.

Rigidity is a bit more subtle. It refers to stiffness of the limbs, which resist movement and have increased inertia. This requires an actual putting on of the hands. I moved his arms slowly. The resistance was there and it had the right quality, as if pulling the arm over a cogwheel. The cogwheel rigidity of Parkinson's disease. So now he had two out of the four. Ain't neurology easy? Like passing a vaginal speculum. Or putting on outlet forceps.

The third aspect of Parkinson's is called bradykinesia; literally this means slow movements and it encompasses a host of symptoms from a poverty of spontaneous movements, to difficulty in initiating movements, to profound slowness of such movements. One of the hallmarks is the classic slow, small, labored handwriting known as micrographia. I had Fred Gould write a few sentences for me. He did and I saw that he had micrographic handwriting. He also had other signs. His arms didn't swing as he walked. His legs shuffled ever so little. There was a decrease in facial movements. His finger movements were slowed, not much, but enough to be abnormal. Three down. All that was missing was the loss of postural reflexes, or imbalance, but that usually is seen only after years of having the disease. Three out of four. Ergo, Parkinson's disease.

I haven't seen Fred Gould since that day and I really didn't ever expect to see him again. Why? It's not a matter of distance. He's flown to New York for medical care. Chicago is no more difficult to get to. He gets on a plane at Zurich and gets off at O'Hare instead of JFK. Not a big deal. It's almost as if we both know it's better this way. We talk once every three or four months. Often about advances in research. Sometimes about his condition. He's the type of patient with whom I do the worst. He's the one who has to be in charge at all times. Who has to make all the decisions based on his own needs at that moment. Patients always make the final decisions. I respect that. It's their absolute right. But they do not have the right to ignore my advice, make decisions of which I do not approve, decisions that I believe are wrong and harmful, and still consider me to be their doctor. Fred Gould is that kind of patient. He does not understand that a doctor-patient relationship requires one doctor and one patient and that he can't be the doctor, since I am not going to be his patient.

So we talk. He's very bright. Exceptionally so. He's from Egypt. But he is not really an Egyptian. He was just born there. He's a Hungarian Jew whose family came to Egypt during the early part of this century, sometime before the First World War and stayed there in business until Nasser took over and then they, like most of the other Jews of Egypt, were forced to leave their homes and businesses and go somewhere else—anywhere else. He and his family ended up in Geneva, in the oil business. The family was not originally in the oil business. I don't remember what they did in Egypt, but Fred is an oil broker. He imports oil into Europe, from Egypt. He has old friends there. Important friends. People he went to school with. The upper crust of Egyptian society, foreign-born, Muslim, Copt all went to school together. In Egypt and then to a European university. Often in Switzerland. Lausanne. One of his old friends became the oil minister. And Fred, in turn, became an oil broker. Fred has contacts everywhere and somehow he learns about things before I do. Like articles in the *L.A. Times*. So check it out for me if you can.

Subject: Brain implants in Parkinson's disease
Place: Mexico City
Name: Garcia. Sandalio Garcia

I'm sure it's just one of those rumors. The Swedes have already done a number of similar procedures in patients with PD. They studied their patients quite carefully. None of their patients improved very much. And they know more about Parkinson's disease than anyone in Mexico City.

Roger

August

The tremor that so distresses patients with Parkinson's disease invariably goes away during sleep, only to return the next morning as soon as the patient awakens. This is a fact, a clinical observation that has been documented thousands and thousands of times. Yet no one knows why this occurs. Each medical student learns this fact when he studies neurology. The inquisitive student recognizes the strangeness of this and asks, "Why does the tremor go away during sleep?" That is not the real issue. During sleep the brain is functioning normally and producing normal behavior. The real problem is to understand why the tremor comes back the next morning.

Harold L. Klawans
Toscanini's Fumble

August 1

Randall Jackson, Esq.
Miksis, Smalley and Cavaretta, P.C.
3600 North Sheffield
Chicago, IL 60651

Dear Randy,

As best as I can tell, the following are the more significant differences between Martin Bloom, presumably living plaintiff, and Marty Bloom, innocent but deceased literary figure as portrayed in *Toscanini's Miscue*. The former will hereafter be known as the real Martin Bloom, although he is no more real than any other Martin Bloom, and were he to admit that the other Martin Bloom is not real, an admission I as an author would never admit to, then there would be no case, which there probably isn't in reality, merely in our courts, which are as divorced from reality as they are from justice. As Justice Oliver Wendell Holmes put it, our courts are courts of law, not of justice. Clarence Darrow said much the same thing, about the courts not being a stage for justice but an arena for opposing lawyers. I quoted him in one of my books. Holmes, not Darrow. Somehow I misidentified him as a Chief Justice of the Supreme Court, not as an Associate Justice, which is what he was. My editor missed that flub, but one reader caught my mistake and wrote me about it. Not very good, considering that when I used the wrong earned run average for some obscure pitcher of little note, six people wrote letters to me. Perhaps that is why the courts are more bankrupt these days than baseball. Hard to believe, isn't it?

Back to justice. The real Martin Bloom was born in Chicago in 1927, at least according to *The Baseball Encyclopedia*. He pitched for the White Sox in 1948, 1949, and 1951. He was apparently somewhere in the minor leagues in 1950. Where, I do not know. *The Baseball Encyclopedia* is silent on such matters. It only gives facts about a player's major league career. I'm certain we can find out. All we need is an old Sporting News *Baseball Register*. He was also in the minors for most of '48 and '49. Where? Memphis is a possibility. That was a Sox farm club then. So was Waterloo. And Colorado Springs, I think. His only full season in the majors was 1951. That year of sainted memory was the year when Paul Richards led us from the doldrums into contention. The other Martin Bloom, the fictionalized character in "The Legacy," one of

34

the essays in *Toscanini's Miscue*, was in high school in the 1950s, when he and I were both White Sox fans cheering for the real Marty Bloom along with Saul Rogovin and all our other heroes. He, the unreal one, was a friend of mine and high school classmate at a time when the real Marty was already out of the big leagues [see page 113 of *Toscanini's Miscue*]. I, of course, cannot tell you his real name. That is privileged information. He was a patient of mine. A real, live patient. Now dead, but still protected. Still privileged.

Please note that all of the other White Sox players mentioned on that same page are mentioned solely in the context of my recalling the 1953 White Sox. I do not know how to reminisce about nameless ballplayers. That is worse than taking the proverbial shower wearing boots or a raincoat. The ones mentioned include Minnie Minoso, Chico Carrrasquel, Virgil Trucks, Billy Pierce, and Nellie Fox. I am, by the way, team physician of the Nellie Fox Society, an honor that I rank as one of the greatest in my medical career. That, however, is another story; one I will certainly not tell here.

Other players are also mentioned in the same sense. The heroes of my youth, fondly recalled: Bob Elliot, Tom Byrne, Paul Richards, and Sandalio Consuegra.

My Martin Bloom was seen by me as a patient in 1974. At that time he was thirty-seven years old. Please note that the real Martin Bloom was forty-seven in 1974. A difference of ten years, but who is counting? Certainly not Martin Bloom. Or his lawyer.

My character had gone to the University of Colorado and then gone into his father's real estate business. There is never any hint at all that my literary character ever played major league baseball. The real Martin Bloom went to the University of Iowa and did play major league baseball. That's what started this all. Why did the Sox ever call him up? They should have left him down in Memphis. Or Colorado Springs. Or Waterloo. With Rocky Krsnick and J.W. Porter, two other minor league players who never really made it.

My character had end-stage renal disease by age thirty-one [1968], had a renal transplant at age thirty-six in 1973, and had been given a polio injection in the kitchen of my home by my father in 1955. As far as I know, the real Martin Bloom was never in the kitchen of my home, never met my father, and was never inoculated by my father for polio. Or anything else. All of those things happened to my character, my patient. My character also died within a few months of the onset of his neurologic disease, that is, in 1974.

THE FOLLOWING AUTHOR'S NOTE SHOULD ALSO BE NOTED
[PAGE 128]:
"I have written about the patient I have called Martin Bloom once
before. He is one of the patients featured in *Sins of Omission*. In
that novel, his symptoms and signs are presented primarily from
the perspective of teaching the art of differential diagnosis." N.B.
"called Martin Bloom."

I hope this is helpful to you. It will save you from having to read my
book. Did the real Martin Bloom read it? Did his lawyer? Did you? Will
you? Are such matters irrelevant? Will the judge? Will his decision
depend on what is actually written in my book?
Can any of the above read? You, of course, excluded.
My Martin Bloom, by the way, was a third cousin of Leopold Bloom.
Tell that to Martin's lawyer. Yes, *the* Leopold Bloom!

> Roger "Doc" Kramer
> Team Physician, Nellie
> Fox Society

cc: Rob

August 2

Dear Rob,
Of course, it's not science fiction. The phrase *brain transplant* conjures up all sorts of peculiar images. Frankenstein. God knows what else.
That's why the popular press uses the term, but what Garcia is doing is
not a brain transplant. No brain is being taken from one patient and then
transplanted into someone else. There is no brain donor and no brain
recipient. No one is pronounced brain-dead. Nothing like that at all. It's
an implant, an adrenal implant. Part of the patient's own adrenal gland
put into the brain.
The process resembles a skin graft more than a transplant. Nothing
more. Tissue from one part of the patient's own body is being grafted
onto another part of his body. Big deal. We've been doing these sorts of
procedures for decades. Skin. Bone. Blood vessels. Isn't a coronary
bypass really a saphenous vein implant? Well, in this procedure part of

the patient's own adrenal gland is put into his brain. You are right: it should be called an adrenal implant. After all, it is the adrenal gland that is being implanted, but the phrase *brain transplant* sells many more newspapers.

The procedure is all very straightforward. I am sure that you do more complicated operations, Rob. It just combines two fairly standard operations. A general surgeon removes one of the patient's two adrenal glands. Nothing fancy in that. General surgeons do it all the time for patients with various forms of cancers, on patients who were a lot sicker than most PD patients.

The adrenal gland, once removed, gets diced up into nice small bits. Sort of like dicing an onion. It's the ability of these little bits to make dopamine that may be the key to the puzzle. In PD the brain has lost its ability to make dopamine. The cells of the adrenal gland have this ability. That's why they are put into the brain; in order to make dopamine exactly at that place in the brain where the PD patients need it. In the meantime, back at the operating table, the neurosurgeon gets the brain ready to receive the implant. Where? Not just any place, but the place where the dopamine is missing, a motor relay station called the striatum. The striatum is where the dopamine isn't in PD. Once the neurosurgeon has found the striatum, he removes a small part of it and then packs the small pieces of the adrenal medulla into the resulting cavity. That's it. The implant procedure is all over. The cells are there. All they have to do now is survive and make dopamine.

But do they survive? Who knows? They don't in most animals. They didn't in the Swedish patients, although their procedure was a bit different.

There are a lot of unanswered questions. Do the adrenal cells survive? Do they make dopamine? It's not what they do best. Or normally. And do the patients get better? That is the question of questions. The only one that matters. The Swedish patients didn't. Rumor has it the Mexican patients did. By the way, thanks for the article.

Fred Gould called again. He's my patient from Geneva. I told him to call me back when Garcia publishes his results in the *New England Journal of Medicine*. Until then, it's just rumor.

On Sunday I stopped by the Chicago Theater Workshop for the first time in a couple of years. They were doing staged readings of three short plays. Works in progress by "playwrights." I used to be very active there, back in the days when I thought I wanted to be a playwright. They do staged readings of plays in progress. The playwright supplies a script and they supply a director, a cast, a simple set, and an audience, mostly other playwrights, actors, friends, and relatives. What follows is a couple of rehearsals and then, on Saturday afternoon, a staged reading. That's what I saw on Saturday. Staged readings of plays in progress. In my mind, they were not making very much progress. And one had to use the term *playwright* very loosely. I never thought of myself as a playwright. Maybe that's why I didn't succeed. I was a novelist trying to write a play or two. There were probably other reasons, too.

I hated all three of the works I saw. Three plays written by people who knew nothing about the theater. Nothing about the tradition. About the works their audiences would already know. Like *You Can't Take It With You*.

Why do people who never read think they can write? That is one of the main differences between science and art, one that is universally ignored. No one really believes he can do world-class scientific research if he or she has not had any scientific training. No one tries to perform research without learning the techniques, without knowledge of the field. No one applies for a federal research grant without first figuring out whether the question they want to answer has already been answered.

But in literature, that's okay. Why not write a short story about some guy who woke up one morning to discover he had been transformed into a giant beetle? What a great idea.

Why do people who know nothing about literature, and appear to have read even less, think they can become serious writers? Somehow they do and it amazes me. Such arrogance. I have never met a scientist who was that arrogant. Is it one of the rights guaranteed by the Constitution? The Bill of Rights? The Fifth Freedom? The right to be creative. Without first paying their dues!

Roger

August 6

Dear Rob,

I just got another call from Geneva. From Fred Gould, of course. I don't know anyone else who would call me from Geneva. "It's in the *New England Journal of Medicine*," he told me.

"What is?" I asked, already guessing that the Mexican rumors had been transformed into scientific facts. The power of the written word. Facts. Data. Science. History. Out of the shadows and into the limelight. On to the Great White Way.

"The article by Garcia, the Mexican neurosurgeon," he said, telling me exactly what I knew I would hear. Confirmation more than information.

"When?" I asked.

"Thursday."

Not the previous Thursday, I quickly learned, but the Thursday that was not yet upon us. And still is not. It being only Tuesday in both Chicago and Geneva, as well as in Mexico City. But Fred had somehow managed to get a pre-print prior to publication. How he had managed that I had no idea, and Fred Gould was not about to tell me. The overall process I understood. The *New England Journal of Medicine* loves making news. In fact, it seems to have become dedicated not just to publishing medical news but also to creating that news. It has become the news. A medical report becomes news because the *NEJM* prints it. That fact makes it news. Makes it important. Makes the rest of the media know that it is important and reliable and valid and newsworthy. If it weren't, would good ol' *NEJM* waste its space? To secure this position, the *NEJM* itself sends out its pre-prints to newspapers, TV stations, and news magazines throughout the world. And apparently, directly or indirectly, to Fred Gould.

"Get me a copy," I requested. In minutes I had one, by fax. I told you faxes were a great thing. After all, you already have the fax of this letter. If I could only fax it to my publisher at the same time. If I had a publisher.

So now I have more than rumors. More than the *L.A. Times*. Real science. Which the *NEJM* has guaranteed to be the best of all possible science.

In the report Garcia describes his treatment of two young patients with supposedly "intractable and incapacitating" Parkinson's disease. Two patients. Only two. I'd heard rumors of more patients than that. So had Fred. And other patients of mine. The procedure was pretty much what I'd understood it to be. More or less what I described to you in my last letter on this matter. Pieces of each patient's own adrenal gland had been transplanted into their brains. The reported results were spectacular. All but beyond belief. Miracles. A trip to Lourdes. Two of them, without Jennifer Jones. Lazarus revisited. It is hard not to get excited. More than hard; it's damn near impossible. I completely understand why Fred called me. In the first patient, all of the features of Parkinson's disease had virtually disappeared within ten months of the operation. The patient had been transformed from a totally immobilized, all but helpless shadow of a man to someone who could play soccer with his twelve-year-old son. Had Lazarus ever played soccer again? I have no idea. When levodopa was first used to treat PD, I had seen such results. It, too, had revolutionized PD. If the implants did as much, they would be mini-miracles.

But one patient does not a revolution make. In the second patient, the same sort of improvement was seen. This time within three months after the operation. Another miracle! A virtual cure!

This is why Fred Gould is so excited. I'm excited and I don't even have PD. But I have patients who do. Hundreds of them. And I need to help them. And the research we are doing now won't cure their disease.

Will this?

It could, but wait. All is not quite what it seems. I'll admit, Rob, I already have my doubts and some of these doubts are because of the source. Call it prejudice. But the fact remains that I have not heard of Garcia or his coauthors and, after all, the last major medical advance to come out of Mexico occurred in 1954, when it was announced that laetrile was *the* cure for cancer. But it isn't just prejudice or skepticism. You know me better than that, Rob. PD is my field. My ballpark. I can read more than what the lines say. The numbers in the article are more than just a scant amount of data. Garcia's article demonstrates a total lack of sophisticated knowledge of Parkinson's disease and its proper evaluation and treatment. You know how the game is played. You read medical journals. Method is damn near everything. And Garcia has no idea what the right methods are. None at all. He didn't use any of the accepted methods of Parkinson's disease research. He has invented his own scale, his own way of evaluating how severe the Parkinson's disease is. Why? There are published scales. Almost every investigator studying Parkinson's disease uses these scales to communicate results, so that the readers actually know what is being described. The neurology journals demand this. Does Garcia even know them? Or does he know as little of PD as the average fledgling playwright does of Kaufman and Hart? Or Kafka? His article shows no evidence that he had ever read the key methods papers. He was as arrogant as those playwrights. Do the editors of *NEJM* know the literature? This is not a trivial question. We're not talking sit-coms here. We're dealing with patients and their lives. Scales are all. Is Garcia's scale valid? Does it really measure what he thinks it does? Accurately? Dependably? Reproducibly? And all the hopes are based on just two patients, one of whom has only been followed for three months. There are just too many unanswered questions.

Or am I just carping? What difference did it make what kind of scale he used? His patients got better. In ways that no scales were designed to measure. Or needed. You can either play soccer or you can't.

Roger

August 9

Dear Rob,

Orwell. You decided to bury yourself in Orwell. *1984, Down and Out in Paris and London, Homage to Catalonia,* and *The Road to Wigan Pier.* I'm sure you'll get to *Burmese Days* and *A Clergyman's Daughter.* What a peculiar choice. Certainly not one that I would have made. Nor even suggested. He was not one of the names I listed in my first letter to you. Why not? That should be obvious. Orwell is a man of ideas. An intellect. A moral genius perhaps. But he is not a stylist. He is not a great novelist. A great thinker—yes. But a mediocre novelist at best. His style is stodgy. He never sinks to the level of mere typing, but he's no Hemingway. It's his ideas that flow, not his words. Not his paragraphs. And not his structure. Nor his development of characters. It works well in his essays but not his novels.

1984 is primarily a tract. A field of ideas. A disturbing, yet brilliant vision of the world. And it is still relevant. And chilling. And, yes, the image of our century is that of a boot stamping down on the face of humanity. He said it better than that. It is his image. But *1984* is not a great novel. It is not just that the world has changed politically. Dostoevski's world is gone, as is Tolstoy's. There are no more czars. The fact is *1984* was never on a par with *War and Peace* as a novel. Nor was *War and Peace* on a par with *1984*.

So, of course, Orwell hated Dali. What choice did he have? None. They are exact opposites. Antipodes, to borrow a phrase. Orwell, a man of vision, a moralist who observed the conditions surrounding humanity, engulfing it, and man's role in producing these conditions, and yet a man with only modest gifts as a writer. What did he see in Dali? The opposite. An artist who was all talent. All technical skill. No humanity. No vision. No morality. What was Orwell's phrase? All of Dali's talent was distal to his elbow? Something like that. And Orwell didn't know the half of it. To him, Dali was an artist without soul. An artist, all of whose talents lay in his arms and hands. A medium without a message.

And Orwell was all message, trying to manipulate his limited medium. Little did Orwell suspect how corrupt Dali's medium would become. But if there is no message, what else can be expected?

In 1971 I visited Mourlot's in Paris. At that time it was the most famous of all the graphic print shops in the world. It still is, I think. They made the lithographs for most of France's master artists. I was there with a Chicago artist named Richard Florsheim. Richard did his lithographs there. In the traditional way. He prepared his own stones. Reworked them. Approved each proof. Each stage. An artist at work. Producing his own lithographs and, once approved, signing them.

Next to Richard was one of the anonymous technicians, drawing images on stones. Big images on big stones. Drawn from a single napkin covered with vague sketches with words like *rouge* and *jaune* scribbled here and there. And from these he produced large flowers and then printed them onto even larger sheets of paper. Sheets of paper already signed. "S. Dali."

Where there is no message, there is no medium. The triumph of corruption.

Are there any fake Dalis? What is real? What is genuine? What are the limits of genuine? What is art? What is merely a reproduction? Why not collect photographs of the Sistine Chapel? We read reports all the time of counterfeit Dalis. The question is whether there are any genuine Dalis.

There are, I suspect, still thousands and thousands of signed sheets of paper, paper of the highest quality, waiting to become original Dalis. The fact that he has been dead for years should hardly be an impediment to his artistic creativity. Orwell must be laughing somewhere.

My agent has received my new novel. Have you seen it on the book racks yet? Have you been in a drugstore? An airport? A newsstand? Your local convenience store? Needless to say, you haven't, and, equally needless to say, my agent loved the novel. Would you like to hear his exact words? Or, more correctly, read them? Do you have a choice? You could always skip to the next page. That's another one of the advantages to letters. You can't skip over parts in a telephone conversation. They only exist in real time. You can't even fast forward them. Back to my agent. He said, and I quote, that my latest novel is:

Brilliant. My best work yet. A sure sell. More taut than anything I've done before. More suspenseful. Worth a far larger advance. Six figures at least. A prime candidate for a combined hardcover/softcover deal.

In other words, the usual response. Why am I so skeptical? I've been there before. More than once. An agent is the first cousin of a used car salesman. There's only one difference. I'm not the buyer; I'm the used car. Or at least *The Blind Observer* is.

I wonder if he read it. He must know it's about AIDS.

So my batting average is on hold. Still .429. No change in either the numerator or the denominator. It's August. Nothing much gets done in publishing in August. Editors, like their shrinks and my agent, leave Manhattan by the droves, so my new novel won't be submitted to any publisher until after Labor Day. So don't run out to a bookstore for a while yet. Or even your local supermarket.

Am I happy with my agent? Do I sound as if I'm not? That, my friend, is a difficult question. I don't know anything about agents. So how did I pick mine? It was easy. I got a list of agents from some medical editors I knew. I called the agents. The calls all went the same way.

I published one novel and had a second novel that I'd finished.

Yawn.

It was a mystery.

Snore.

Set in a hospital.

No response.

My first book had been a Book-of-the-Month Club alternate.

"We'll represent you."

Sight unseen?

Yes.

Book unread? What a ridiculous question. Being a literary agent isn't about reading books. It's about selling books.

So how did I choose my agent? It was easy. I figured I needed someone I could talk to, a baseball fan. But not a Yankee fan. My agent's a Mets fan. Perfect. After all, I cheer for two teams, the White Sox and whoever is playing the Cubs. And eighteen times a year that's the Mets. Believe it or not, that's how I picked him. And who says life does not imitate the World Series?

Roger

August 14

Dear Rob,

David just left my office. He is hobbling far less than he was last week. The pain from his gouty left big toe is obviously better. As David himself pointed out to me, gout always goes away. That is the natural history of the disease. So David's level of pain is less, but not his level of distress. That has increased a dozen-fold. So many people are angry at him. Not just his own doctor; but so many other doctors. His friends. It is a rejection that has left him stunned.

Why, he wonders, are they all so mad at him? What had he done to them? He hadn't rejected their advice. They weren't his doctors. They were bystanders in the issue of his medical care.

"But you rejected them," I told him. "Each and every one of them, as openly as if you, publicly, had thrown a gauntlet at their feet."

"How?" he asked. And it was an honest question. He really did not know. Sometimes I forget that he is not a physician.

I tried to explain it to him without sounding like a condescending physician, like all those other physicians. Most physicians consider themselves to be "treating" physicians. Not observers. But active "treaters." They take care of sick people and cure disease. Or at least that is what they attempt to do. To them, that's what medicine is all about. Not diagnosis, but the treatment of patients. They are special because they treat people. Relieve suffering. Save lives. Stamp out disease. And they have come to believe that that is the way the world is and why they deserve a special place in that world, a world made up of sickness and healers. And they are the healers.

They are wrong. That is not the only perspective. It is certainly the traditional one. Healing isn't the only basis of medicine. Not really. And certainly not for me. Or David. Medicine long antedates any effective treatment of anything. And just because a patient has an untreatable disease, that doesn't mean he is outside the field of medicine. Medicine is the study of diseases. And of patients with diseases. And their care. And care and treatment are not the same thing.

David knows all that. And believes it. And understands it. Perhaps even better than I do because he is not even a part of a patient-physician relationship that can trap the physician, as much as it does the patient, into a predetermined role.

Not so most "treating" physicians. Perhaps that was true during medical school, but not when you're grown up and taking care of sick people. Medicine is treatment. And David had rejected treatment and instead chose to live out and observe the natural history of his self-limited disease.

He had rejected them, each and every one of them. He had rejected the very basis of their lives, their professional commitment, their livelihoods. Of course they were mad at him. What he'd done was a personal affront to each of them, a personal slap in the face. A gauntlet to which there was no reply. No seconds. No duel at dawn. The challenge was an attack. One they could neither answer nor ignore.

"But is treating what it's all about?" he asked me.

"It is the myth that we've sold for the last seventy years or more. The public has bought it. Medicine has even bought it. Observation is what it's really about. Observation and diagnosis. Not treatment. But if that's true, you can't charge three thousand dollars for a carotid artery bypass that takes no longer than a two hundred dollar neurologic consultation."

"They don't."

"Who?"

"The cardiovascular surgeons. They don't charge three grand. They charge five grand."

Nice irony there. The editor ought to like that.

"Perhaps they are right to be angry with you. What would happen if more people with vascular disease opted for the natural history of their disease? After all, most carotid bypasses are being done on patients who probably do not need them. In patients for whom such bypass procedures have yet to be proven to change the final outcome, except, of course, for those patients who have a stroke during surgery, or don't even survive to get off the table."

"How often does that happen?" he asked.

"In the best of hands, one to two percent."

"And in ours?"

"Don't ask."

45

No irony there at all. Just arrogance and the assumption of authority. Routine surgical skills.

David thought for a moment, "But I'm not saying that other people should change what they are doing. I'm just not taking medicine for my gout. It's my big toe that hurts," David protested. "I'm not putting up the barricades."

"They don't know that."

Roger

August 16

Dear Rob,

I've been thinking about Orwell. I'm not so certain that it was merely Dali's corrupt facility, his talent without vision, that was the basis of Orwell's disgust. Orwell was a man who had a faith, a vision, a commitment. Dali had no commitment. Except to himself. Self-indulgence *über alles*. Orwell went to Spain. He fought in the Spanish Civil War. He fought for something he believed in. He fought against Franco. Against Fascism. He stood up and was counted.

What did Dali do? He fled in the other direction. As fast as he could. He made no commitment. He chose neither side but his own. He went to France. He settled in Bordeaux. Good food. Good wine. An easy place to flee from if the war were finally to erupt. And when it did, he did. To where? Spain, then the United States.

But still no commitment.

Orwell judges by that. Not by the dexterity that went no higher than his elbow. Dali's, that is. That was the phrase, I think.

Do artists have to be committed?

A good question. There are some issues that cannot be ignored. The Holocaust. The Spanish Civil War. Racism. Some truths that must be faced.

It is interesting that my interest in visual art comes as a surprise to you. I collected art while we were interns. Not very actively, true, but who had time to do anything very actively? But not knowing that about me shows the nature of what we shared together, the aspects of our bonding. God, I hate that phrase and all it represents. Bonding. Pop psychology. Pseudo-insights. Right brain. Left brain. Neurology for the non-neurologists who prefer not to be confused by data.

Then I collected French art. The School of Paris. Lithographs and etchings. I bought them by mail from Paris.

Who? The obligatory big names: Giacometti. Braque. Laurens. Ernst. Leger. And even some of the second class cubists like Lhote, Severini, and Picabia. And the French abstractionists, who are still unknown in the United States today: Atlan, Bissiere . . . why list the others?

But that was then. Times have changed. I have changed. But not my love for visual art and my need to surround myself with it. The artists whose works I now collect are called Imagists. The Chicago Imagists. A far cry from the abstractionists of my youth. And what they do is create images. They make no claim on reality. They are not creating impressions of a moment. No Sunday afternoons on Oak Street Beach. Not the expression of a single moment of pent-up emotion. Nothing gestural in their art. No screams either. Not the narrative of life and death at its most romantic. No Rafts of the Medusa.

They create images. With capital I's. Bright, bold images. Canvas is canvas. Flat is flat and that flatness, that lack of reality, that has become what art is all about. That and color. Paint is paint. You want the world, the precise moment. The meaning. The expression. The narrative. Take a picture. Get out your camcorder. Watch TV news, where images and news fuse to present us with neither a meaningful image nor real news. If there is no image to present, the event is only worth twenty seconds. If there is, let the cameras click away. Except they don't click anymore. News is news. Its importance has nothing to do with camera work. Tell that to a TV producer.

The ten o'clock news ain't art. The two should never be confused.

But the Imagists are art. And the art they are about are images. Not a reproduction of the world. But of an image of a world of artistic truth.

Who are they? The real question is why have you not heard of them. The answer is simple. American art history is written by New Yorkers. New York art critics. New York curators. The MOMA. As if it is the only Museum of Modern Art. Modern art history is written by Frenchmen with an occasional Italian and German thrown in. So Munch is a nonentity. And the only important Russian is Chagall. And it's all true because it is all that we know. Well, the Imagists are not from New York. They are from Chicago. Not Joe DiMaggio. Not Lou Gehrig. Not Mickey Mantle.

More like Luke Appling. He, too, is in the Hall of Fame. The only shortstop to lead the American league in batting. And he did it twice.

One of them is Roger Brown. Mostly he paints what might be called landscapes, but they are not landscapes in any traditional sense. Often they are city scenes. But it's not everyone's reality that he depicts. To many, it's not even a real vision of the world. After all, the United States is not a flat map covered by an endless succession of identical strip malls. Can that be what artists see when they look at our beautiful country? Have you looked lately? Have they?

And Temple Mount in Jerusalem. That's not a football stadium resting majestically between staged events played out only for the world's TV cameras. Of course not. Go there and see. All those riots you see on the evening news are staged. Rehearsed. Cued. On camera. No camera, no demonstration.

Ed Paschke. He's perhaps the best known of them all. He's had shows at major museums around the world. He gives us the image on our own faulty TV screen. The image is right there, but it's not quite right. It's fuzzy. It's made up of dots. Not dots out of Seurat. Dots out of Sony. Dots that create an image that can never be as clear as it should be. An image that is not quite doubled. Repeated. Blurred. Not clear. Not sharp. Just bright and indelible. And creating true twentieth century icons. Tattooed ladies. Hairy shoes. Everyman. No man. Michael Jordan. M.J. as a bust. Shades of Julius Caesar and all the little Caesars. S.P.Q.R. Transplanted to Chicago. S.P.Q.C.

Paschke and Brown are the most famous, but the list doesn't end with them. It just starts there. There's Christina Ramberg. She has painted a succession of sinister women trussed up in garments half out of Frederick's of Hollywood and half out of your neighborhood leather shop. No one dresses like that. No one you know could be half that bizarre. Or menacing. Yet those stores all stay in business. And not even Joe McCarthy could still believe that they are part of a pinko-commie plot to undermine the American family. She, I am told, no longer paints. She can't. She has Pick's disease. Alzheimer's, only worse. No one can paint with severe Pick's or Alzheimer's. Not even deKooning could do that, even though he didn't have to create images. Despite what his dealers might claim while trying to sell works that he supposedly "painted" while otherwise demented. What a lot of drivel. The problem with global dementia is that it is global.

Then there's Karl Wirsum—the worst of them all. He tries to see humor in it all. Humor in life. Is there any humor in Michelangelo? Or Rembrandt? Or Cézanne? Can you stand in front of a Cézanne and laugh? Or even smile? Hell, no. It's great art he is creating. If he could have smiled, he might have gone to his mother's funeral. *Could*, I wrote, not *would*. Heaven forbid.

You can smile at a Renoir. That can't be real art. I remember a remark I heard Jean Renoir make once. He'd been asked to compare his father and Cézanne. Cézanne, he said, loved apples. His father loved women. And children. And life. And his family. You can even be made to feel relaxed and at peace by a Renoir. But laugh? Karl Wirsum. Every time. What junk. Not real art. Art is not to entertain you. Not to make you feel good.

Then what the hell is it for? To make you understand the seriousness of life, the potential tragedy. Watch a UNICEF ad on TV. Or if one day by mistake the TV news manages to slip in ten seconds of children starving in Somalia or Bangladesh or wherever they are starving that day instead of interviewing a passenger delayed at O'Hare by a snow storm, instead of real news.

Well, life includes laughter. Why can't art? Karl Wirsum says it can. He should have learned the lesson of George S. Kaufman. Comedy keeps the theaters full, but only tragedy is considered to be art. That was not true in ancient Greece. The Greeks thought that Aristophanes was a great playwright.

And I, like the artists whose work I collect, try to create images. Not all of life. Not *War and Peace*. Perhaps the sweep of my vision is limited. Perhaps almost as limited as my skill. But I do have a vision.

Roger

August 22

Dear Rob,

We are just about ready to get into the implant business. Our neurosurgeon, Frank Fain, visited Sandalio Garcia in Mexico City. According to Fain, who has visited a lot of neurosurgeons in his day, Garcia was up-front with him. Everything was out in the open. He showed Frank his patients and even had him watch him perform an implant. Frank is quite certain that he can do the exact procedure without any problems. That, of course, is what we want to do, what we need to do, in order to completely evaluate Garcia's exact procedure. Not re-do what the Swedes dia, reproduce what Garcia is doing. That, after all, is the real question. Does his procedure, the Garcia implant technique, done the way he does it, really help patients with Parkinson's disease? His technique, but done on our patients. Patients with known PD that has been diagnosed, treated, and evaluated by experts on Parkinson's disease, using the right scales, speaking the right scientific language. The gauntlet has been thrown. And we are responding. Scientifically. Carefully. As detached scientists. Believe that and I'll sell you a bridge or two. Of course we are doing it scientifically. That is what we are. We are medical scientists. We know the game. We are the game. But we are not detached. It's exciting. And we are in the middle of that excitement. Maybe not Columbus exactly, but Henry Hudson. At least.

We have submitted our protocol to the hospital's Committee on Human Investigation, so now we must sit and wait. How long will that take? For a brain implant? Who knows? We've been fighting with them for three months about a study on the effect of diet on PD. We don't want to change anyone's diet. No restrictions. No additives. All we want to do is rearrange the total amount of protein in the diet. Rearrange, not change. Very little protein for breakfast. Very little at lunch. A lot at supper. And that debate has been going on for three months. A succession of questions. Of arguments. Of t's to dot and i's to cross. Or vice versa. Or both. Call it research.

Others have already started doing the procedure. One is George Baumer. He's a neurosurgeon in Ann Arbor. In fact, he's head of neurosurgery there. That is a real medical center. Baumer is the first one in the United States to do an adrenal implant, replete with TV news conferences and an article in *Time* magazine. It's the Jerusalem question again. If there were no cameras, would he have wanted to be first? No press conferences. Not Christian Barnard revisited. Not heart transplants recreated. Just plain old-fashioned science. Neurosurgeons from all over the country are all jumping on the bandwagon. Even places that have no expertise in Parkinson's disease. And no experience. That is not a good combination, believe me. Parkinson patients with severe disease are fragile. Things can go wrong. They do. All the time. And patients can die. So damn easily. From what? Anything. Often we don't even know why. Even in places like Memphis. You remember Memphis? That's where Marty Bloom pitched when he wasn't pitching in Chicago. The Memphis Chicks.

Did you see the article in the *New York Times*? It came out three or four days ago. So far I've received a couple of dozen copies. Some were brought in by patients, others were mailed to me. A couple came in by fax. One of those came from Geneva, of course. The article is about Garcia and his technique. "His technique." That's why we have to do what he did. All in all, it's a rave review. My books should only get such good reviews. They called Garcia's accomplishment a miracle. Does that make him a saint? Or just a pre-saint? A saint-in-waiting? Like a play in progress. I guess that's as close to official canonization as he can get. This side of Stockholm. Or Rome. They interviewed Garcia and also several of his patients in Mexico City. They certainly have jumped on Garcia's bandwagon. And why shouldn't they? Beware the rhetorical question. We're getting half a dozen phone calls a day or more from patients we've never even seen. The *New York Times* was more than enthusiastic. They were downright orgasmic. They believed Garcia. And all his claims. Why not? He told them that most of his eighteen patients were almost cured!

Most of the eighteen patients! The *New York Times* can count. Two could be flukes, but eighteen! That's a real number. Not just a couple of statistical outriders, but eighteen patients. No wonder they were so orgasmic. It was this number that made believers of them and the whole world of patients and media. Garcia had now been sanctified by both the *New England Journal* and the *New York Times*. Rome and Constantinople. Or Rome and Jerusalem. But where had all those patients come from?

Many of us doubted that he had only operated on those two patients he picked to write up for the *NEJM* article. But even the rumors we'd heard had not included this many patients. Eighteen implants. And there were far more than just two successes. It cannot be written off as a couple of flukes. Something was happening. Something important. The enthusiasm is contagious. It is unlike anything I've seen or felt since the early days of levodopa, the first real breakthrough in the treatment of Parkinson's disease. That was over twenty years ago. It's been a long time between breakthroughs. Slowing progression of the disease is good. It's more than good. But it doesn't make people feel better.

It doesn't cure them. It doesn't stamp out their disease. But now the next miracle could be upon us. The patients all want it. They need it. They deserve it. And we want to give it to them. Make no mistake about that. We may need it just as much as they do, want it just as much. So we'll do implants.

And while we're at it, we'll try to answer some scientific questions. How often does it work? If it fails, how often? And why? But what the hell is really going on in Mexico City? It's hard to avoid that question. Where had the other patients suddenly come from? When had they been operated on? Before the *NEJM* article? After? During? All of the above?

What had happened to those who had not been cured? This was the only question the *Times* had asked. Three had died. Three out of eighteen. .167. Better than I ever hit. When? Two, it seems, had died before the *NEJM* article had been published. What ever happened to scientific truth? He'd had as many deaths as the two successes he'd published.

Fred called again. He wants an implant. Who doesn't? He'd like to have it here. He is my patient, he said. I told him we haven't started yet. I told him to call back. He will. You can bet the house on that.

Roger

August 26

Dear Rob,

I was not belittling Martin Bloom's accomplishments. Would I ever do such a thing? God forbid. He was one of my boyhood heroes. I loved him. He was bigger than life. A Jewish kid playing for the White Sox and helping to beat the Yankees. David against Goliath. More real to me than Michelangelo's *David* would ever be. He had been a great high school athlete in Chicago. That didn't matter so much. It was beating those Yankees. I don't remember if he ever really did. No matter. Symbolically he did. And it was his symbolic meaning that mattered. Pitcher as metaphor. Before Susan Sontag. If my memory serves me well, which it usually does, except in the matter of names, he was an All-American pitcher at the University of Iowa. I even believe that some of his collegiate pitching records still stand, almost fifty years later. Not bad. Most of Jesse Owens' records didn't last that long. Nor Babe Ruth's sixty home runs in a single season. Although his record of consecutive shutout innings in the World Series did. But as a major league pitcher, Martin Bloom, the real Martin Bloom that is, would have had to turn it up a few notches to be mediocre. Yes, I do know precisely what mediocre means. Do you? I already am a writer. I use a dictionary all the time. And not just for spelling. And a thesaurus. Roget's. He, too, was a physician.

I've checked Marvelous Marty's record with the baseball encyclopedia. Mediocre means average. Is this an average career? These are all the gory details of that entire major league career.

Games Pitched In: 45. That's total games. All the games he ever got into in the big leagues.

Wins: 5.

Losses: 3.

Win-Loss Percentage: .625. Better than my publishing average. That I grant you. Or do I? Every game has a winning pitcher. And a losing pitcher. One win. One loss. Fifty percent. That's what happens in each game, so that the league win-loss percentage is always fifty percent. .500. Every year. But there is no expected fifty percent for all novelists. It could be zero. .000. I have friends who have written novels and are batting .000. Like Bill Wight's batting average. He was one of the Sox great young lefties. He once went zero for fifty-six. .000.

Innings Pitched: 84 and 2/3. That's all the innings he ever pitched in the big leagues. In his entire career. At nine innings per game, that's only eight complete games, but no one pitches complete games anymore.

Strikeouts: 34.

Strikeouts Per Nine Innings: 3.6.

Walks: 58.

Per Nine Innings: 6.15. Ain't baseball great? More statistics than any research project I ever designed. More than even a sophisticated biostatistician could dream up. And with such great acronyms. And what's more, the numbers are real, unlike the numbers in the publishing industry. Unlike the way paperback sales are calculated. Do you know how that's done? Don't ask; you don't really want to know.

Strike Out/Walk Ratio: .58. One is considered mediocre.

Hits Surrendered: 85.

Hits Per Nine Innings: 1.00.

Why go on? He only won five lousy games in his entire career. And I'm certain he never beat the Yankees. Some David. He's more like Delilah.

Cutting off what little hair I have left.

Roger

August 30

Dear Rob,

I went to a Cubs game this afternoon. I had no choice in the matter. I went with everyone from the lab. We try to go to one baseball game a year and I had missed the last couple of years and Paul Carvey—he runs the lab—thought I ought to go this year. Team unity, you know.

I agreed. What the hell. After all, Paul did get me a seat to the White Sox play-off game in '83 against Baltimore. Such acts should never be forgotten. Even though we lost the game.

So we all went. Lab techs, research scientists, grad students. A real combination. In so many ways. One grad student is from Taiwan. One originally from Viet Nam. One is from India. Not exactly a group of old southsiders who grew up in the shadow of Comiskey Park. I'm sure none of them ever heard of Marty Bloom. Or Sandy Koufax, for that matter. We had upper deck box seats, high up between home plate and first base. In good ol' Wrigley Field. Or, to put it more correctly, "The Friendly Confines of Wrigley Field." I hadn't been inside those confines in a decade. And it always seems strange to me. Foreign. Wrong. It's not Comiskey Park. It's foreign territory. Do I have my passport? Are my immunizations up to date? Can you drink the water? What water? It's a ball park.

How about the Cokes?

Then it hit me. It wasn't all that strange, that unfamiliar, that foreign. Déjà vu. I'd sat there once before. In those exact same seats. I had been there before. I remembered how the field looked from this angle. Once before, but a long time ago. Déjà vu all over again. I tried hard to recall precisely when. Then it hit me. It had been 1949.

Why had I been there? Another good question. My mother had taken me to see a baseball game. A Cubs game, no less. By '49 I was a confirmed Sox fan. Or addict. I hated the Cubs. They were the enemy. The Cubs and the Yankees. I wasn't certain then which was worse. I rooted for three teams. The Sox, whoever was playing the Cubs, and whoever was facing the Yankees. In that order. I cheered for Martin Bloom. Not Bill Nicholson. Or Eddie Waitkus. Or Bob Rush. Or Hank Sauer.

My mother did not hate the Cubs. She disliked every baseball team equally. The whole sport bored her to distraction. It was a taste she'd never acquired. Opera, yes. Even Wagner. But not baseball. So why had we gone to that game? Why had she taken me and a friend? To a Cubs game?

And then for the first time in my life, I knew.

We hadn't gone to a Cubs game. The Cubs just happened to be the home team that day. We had gone to see the Brooklyn Dodgers. Not the Cubs. The Dodgers and their star. We'd gone to Wrigley Field to see Jackie Robinson.

It was, as far as I know, the only baseball game my mother ever went to, at least in my lifetime. And she'd even told me why. It just hadn't really registered.

"You should see Jackie Robinson play," she'd said to me.

"And Ted Williams," I added, "and Stan Musial, and maybe even Joe DiMaggio." Even though he played for the Yankees. The Yankee Clipper.

"Jackie Robinson," she repeated.

And we did. And the Dodgers won. Robinson got two hits. He stole a base. The place was packed.

I saw Williams play a couple of dozen times. Musial half a dozen. DiMaggio three times. And Robinson only that once, but until Paul Carvey made me go back to Cubs Park, I hadn't thought about that game for over forty years.

My parents were not liberals by any means. But mom always knew what was right and tried hard to teach me. And Jackie being in the big leagues was right.

As I sat down that day to watch the Phillies beat the Cubs, I kept remembering the old Dodgers and wiping an occasional tear from my eye. My mom died six years ago and I couldn't call to tell her that I finally understood.

Roger

September

Niels Bohr, the brilliant twentieth century atomic physicist, had a horseshoe nailed to the wall of his house. Other scientists were scandalized by this behavior; they could not believe that Bohr accepted such superstitions. He always replied that he didn't. "But," he would add, "I've been told they work even if you don't believe in them."

Harold L. Klawans
Newton's Madness

September 3

Dear Rob,

It is not that peculiar that I am hesitant to give you specific advice or even general rules to create by. This is not a course in creative writing. And besides, all such advice when put down on paper does not seem so utterly profound. The line that separates sheer buffoonery from profundity becomes narrow and treacherous and may not even exist; it is a boundary that exists more in the eye of the beholder than in reality. Rilke, you remember Rilke. Have you read any Rilke yet? Or even looked him up in the *World Book Encyclopedia*? Right there, between Riley and Rimbaud. Or did you get sidetracked by one of the others? Rimbaud, I hope. Then you can get into Mallarmé and all that symbolist stuff. Does anyone still read Riley? Even in Indiana? Does anyone still wear a hat? Or spats?

Back to Rilke. He wrote a set of letters to a young poet, known to posterity as his *Letters to a Young Poet*. In one of those letters, Rilke urged the young poet—to whom he was writing from Paris or Viareggio or Rome, but somewhere that conjures up images more creative and far more romantic, that's the key word here, romantic, more romantic than Chicago— Rilke urged this all but unnamed poet to look into his own soul at the most quiet hour of his night and not to seek the advice of others but to discover his own nature and his own essence and to write from that essence within the vastness of his own solitude. Orwell looked into his own soul. Not just in the middle of the night, but twenty-four hours a day. Perhaps to a point where it impeded his art. He looked. He saw. He felt his soul.

Dali had none. The old saw that the difference between Dali and an insane man was that Dali was crazier is wrong. The difference is that Dali lacked sincerity. And soul. Psychosis is always sincere. Otherwise it is not psychosis. Psychotics are psychotic to the base of their souls.

Rilke knew that talent without soul was bogus. He gave the poet this simple advice. Not in those words. He was Rilke. He did it in letters that were all so well crafted, so well put together that they made his advice, his everyday admonitions, profound. Even enduring.

But you and I have already looked into our souls at two in the morning when there was nowhere else to look, no one else to turn to, and the patient was going down the tubes, dying right in front of us. We looked. And I think each of us found what we each needed. If we hadn't, we'd have become radiologists. One of our cohorts did. Or pathologists. Or hospital administrators. We didn't. We still take care of sick people.

So, of course, we, having looked into our souls, might think that writing, writing from the soul, is easy. A cinch. It ain't. It's not the same soul.

"This above all, to thine own self be true," said Polonius. Or Shakespeare speaking through Polonius. Not quite so profound. Although perhaps better crafted and undoubtedly more enduring. "Neither a borrower nor a lender be," they went on. Shakespeare and Polonius. No one takes Polonius seriously. He is given to us by actors and directors as a sort of buffoon. A doddering old man at best. But was he? Read Medawar's *Advice to a Young Scientist*. He won a Nobel Prize in chemistry. Medawar, not Polonius. He takes Polonius at his word. Words that should be taken seriously. But Medawar is a scientist, not an actor. Letting actors interpret the word may be very dangerous. Almost as dangerous as letting scientists do it.

Rilke, in one of those letters, the same letter I think, also told the young poet the names of those two books that he never traveled without, those two monumental works that were, to him, unending sources of inspiration, of understanding, guides to getting in touch with his own wellsprings of artistic creativity.

Any guesses? Shakespeare? Dante? How about Homer? Keats? Shelley? Why not Goethe? Rilke wrote in German. Or Heine? The greatest of all German lyric poets. Or Schiller? He wrote *William Tell* and much else that no one reads today.

None of the above.

The Bible was one. Okay, I'll buy that. And Jacobsen.

Who?

Jacobsen. A Scandinavian writer whose works are essentially unobtainable in English today. A Dane. J. P. Jacobsen. And this was the one author Rilke advised him to read, to study, to digest, to incorporate into his soul and being. Not Shakespeare. Not even Goethe. Jacobsen. Rilke felt that Jacobsen was as great a creative being as Auguste Rodin, the French sculptor and "the greatest of all living artists." An interesting judgment, that. It was 1903. What about Monet? The water lilies were yet to come, but the haystacks were there. And the Cathedrals of Rouen. And the London scenes.

Van Gogh was dead. So were Gauguin and Seurat. But Picasso was painting away, in Paris, not far from Rilke. To say nothing of Cézanne. Rilke had yet to see a single Cézanne. Did Rilke and Picasso ever meet? Did Lenin and Joyce when they were living in Switzerland during the Great War?

So I won't tell you what books you should read. I hardly know what I should be reading. But Rilke did give that poet some good advice. Be certain that you really need to be a writer, an artist, a poet. Take that advice. Look into your soul, at two in the morning, at one of those times that remind you of your internship. A quiet time. A time to look into the vastness of your own solitude—that's not a bad phrase. You can a borrower be. So much for Polonius. At one of those times when you are in touch with yourself. Like the time you decided to go into ob/gyn. And this time ask yourself if you need to be a writer. Is expression the need of your soul?

It is of mine. And I'm not certain I know why. And once you know the answer, you will find subjects to write about everywhere. Your childhood. Your home life. Your patients. Your colleagues. Your employers. Your receptionist. Even your billing clerks.

Rilke, in another letter, wrote that he could not send the poet any of his books. He could not afford to. Once his books were published, he wrote, they no longer belonged to him. That remark is true in more ways than merely economics. While it is being written, the book is mine. It is me. My heart. My soul. My libido. My ego. I live it and I breathe it. Then the book changes. Not just because of editorial tampering. Editors are a nuisance. A bother. Ravens pecking at your liver. But it's still your liver.

Then someone else picks out a cover. There is that wonderful scene in Graham Greene's *The Third Man*. Our hero, Rollo Martins, meets a friend of Harry Lime's at a cafe; the friend is carrying one of his books, and opens the conversation by complimenting Martins on the cover. The cover! It catches the spirit so well. It's not Martins' cover. The cover never is. The publisher hires some artists to design a cover. I sometimes get to see the cover before the marketing people, but only sometimes. And once that cover exists, it is no longer my book. It no longer occupies my soul. It has become decathected. Detached. Severed. Amputated. I also do not pick the paper, the size, the format, the type, the cover quotes, the picture. Only the words, and by the time they appear they are old. From a past era. Yesterday's box score. Last year's mistress.

Mulisch. Harry Mulisch. There, I've broken my own rule. *The Assault* by Harry Mulisch. It's the best book I've read in the last five or six years. I've read it four times. And read *Amadeus*. Once. Both are more readily available than anything by Jacobsen. Whoever he was.

Roger

September 4

Dear Rob,

I was in Indianapolis yesterday lecturing on Parkinson's disease. The official title of my talk was "Recent Advances in Parkinson's Disease." What else? I've been giving different lectures with that same title for twenty-four years now. It has to be time to quit. Or change the title. Recent setbacks perhaps?

I drove down. It's faster than flying. It takes over an hour just to get from my place to O'Hare. And only two and a half hours to drive to Indianapolis. On the way I listened to a taped version of John Updike's *S*. The novel must be a couple of years old by now. He's completed at least one Rabbit book since *S*. *Rabbit Revisited*. Or *Rabbit III*. I forget. The tape was shorter than I figured it would be. Severely bowdlerized, I'm sure. It finished as I got there. So I decided that since I had half an hour to spare I'd find a bookstore and pick up another audio book to listen to on the way home. I drove to the nearest strip mall. That mall was right out of a Roger Brown oil painting. So was the one across the street. The one I drove in to was the epitome of an American strip mall. It out-"Browned" Roger. A strip mall par excellence. You know the type, complete with a Wal-Mart, a grocery store, forgive me, a supermarket, a Payless Shoes, two or three clothing stores, a store that sells weight loss as best as I could tell, and two video stores. No bookstores.

On to the next mall. Same as the first. Only the names were changed to protect the innocent. Or trap the unwary. Wal-Mart became K-Mart. Blockbuster Video became West Coast Video. Or vice versa. It's hard for me to tell them apart. Kroger became Jewel Foods or vice versa. Wendy's became Burger King. Who even cares which is which? Baker's Square became Denny's. Pizza Hut became Domino's. There was only one constant. No bookstore. None at all.

Another mall. Back to Wal-Mart. Kroger, Wendy's, Baker's Square. Pizza Hut. And no bookstores. Roger Brown's artistic vision is correct. The landscape of the United States is forty-eight contiguous states covered by identical strip malls. And all with *no bookstores*.

Why write a novel? Nobody will read it. No one can. If you can't even find a bookstore, how the hell can you buy a book? Write a screenplay. All the strip malls have video stores. At least one. Often two or three.

My lecture was sponsored by Sandoz. They now distribute Eldepryl for Mylan. As part of my talk I told the story of Eldepryl. It is a triumph of capitalism. Good ol' entrepreneurial capitalism. Not the development of the drug itself. The drug is an old drug. It was developed in Hungary in the 1950s and has been available in Europe since that time, and never used very much. It was developed as an antidepressant. And it is, but not a very good one. Not good enough that anyone ever wanted to try to sell it in the United States, the world's biggest pharmaceutical marketplace. But in the early 1980s there was a young chemist in California, near San Jose. He was a classic American small businessman. An entrepreneur par excellence. Actually, not that excellent. He was very good at marketing and distribution. Those were the secrets of his success. He was not so good at manufacturing. What this chemist did, in his own home, was make what he thought was Demerol to distribute to his friends, neighbors, relations, or anybody else who was addicted to narcotics. The problem is that what he made was not Demerol. It was a Demerol analog, a closely related chemical. And this Demerol analog may have unlocked the secret of Parkinson's disease. Hundreds of people bought it. I told you he was good at marketing and distribution. And at least seven of them came down with severe Parkinson's disease within days to weeks. Seven young addicts with severe Parkinson's disease. Just like that. What a breakthrough!

It was Bill Langston, a neurologist from that area, who first realized how important a discovery this was. Soon after it was shown that the specific chemical that had been brewed up was a chemical related to Demerol. It is now known as MPTP. When this chemical is injected into virtually any animal, it causes that animal to become severely parkinsonian within days. And the brains of that animal shows the exact same changes as we see in the brains of patients with Parkinson's disease. So this so-called "degenerative" disease might not be so degenerative. It might be the result of a toxic exposure. And then came about another brilliant discovery. If you pre-treat an animal with an enzyme inhibitor, like Eldepryl, a drug that blocks the breakdown of MPTP into its more active breakdown product, the animal does not become parkinsonian when you give it MPTP. Eldepryl prevents the disease. Or at least an animal model of a disease. Prevents it. Stamps it out. What a phenomenon! What potential! Let's assume Parkinson's disease is toxic, and that there is some toxin floating around the world that must be converted by this enzyme into its active component. And that's what causes Parkinson's disease and makes it progress.

Could we then stop that progression? That's what the Parkinson Study Group was all about. A number of us came together for two years and designed the experiments, spent another six months writing up the application to try to get the federal government to underwrite it, and then, in the largest clinical experiment ever done in Parkinson's disease, found eight hundred Parkinson patients, gave half of them Eldepryl and the other half various placebos, and looked to see what happened. And it appears that what happened was that the disease did not progress as much in those who received Eldepryl.

Is that the whole story? We never tell the whole story. We never have the whole story. It's like any great piece of literature. Do you know the whole story of Hamlet? Hell, no. Did Fortinbras make a good king? Were the people of Denmark better off under Hamlet's father or Claudius? And why the hell did Gertrude help Claudius kill her husband? Merely because Claudius was ambitious and they were screwing? Or was Hamlet's father a wife-abuser who left her with no other choice? He sure as hell produced an indecisive passive-aggressive son who had visual and auditory hallucinations. All we know are the indecisions of Hamlet and his final action. Murder. Coupled with maternal suicide. Bodies everywhere. But hardly the whole story!

But I digress.

Where does that leave us now? Our hypothesis was that Eldepryl, when given early in the course of Parkinson's disease, would delay the progression of the disease such that patients would not require standard therapy as quickly. The data supported that hypothesis. That's it! It didn't disprove it! That's what data does. It proves nothing. It can disprove a hypothesis, but it can't prove one to be true. Science at work. But was this effect due to slowing the progression of the disease? Or did Eldepryl somehow have a mild beneficial effect, a therapeutic effect, so that all we were doing was actually treating the disease a little bit? I guess that's possible, but all our data and everything our biostatisticians have told us suggest that that is not true. Besides, that's not the only data that Eldepryl does something. There is European data that says patients on Eldepryl who have Parkinson's disease live longer than other parkinsonian patients who were not on Eldepryl.

That's what we're doing these days in Parkinson's disease. That plus implants. And I told the audience these stories and talked about the use of Eldepryl and how to use Sinemet and how to use the other newer drugs in the treatment of Parkinson's disease, and drove back home not listening to any book at all. *S*, by the way, is an epistilatory novel. I'm into reading epistilatory novels these days. After all, I'm writing one. I've reread *You Know Me, Al* by Ring Lardner, read *Wake Up, Stupid* by Mark Harris, and listened to *S* by John Updike. I read it two or three years ago. So far I have not gotten up the enthusiasm to take on *Pamela* by Richardson. That was supposedly the first true novel in the English language and it was written in the form of letters. I'll probably try *The Late George Aply* first.

Sincerely

Roger

P.S. By the way, did you know that Bowdler, the one who became an adjective, was a physician? He, however, gave up medicine. He apparently couldn't stand the sight of blood. Today, he could have become a psychiatrist and censored his patient's dreams. Better than rewriting *Lear.*
So was Rabelais.

September 7

Dear Rob,

Of course you had no idea I had been writing plays. There was no way you could, living as you do some two thousand miles from Chicago. I do not consider myself to be a playwright. After all, no one has ever produced a play of mine. For a while, I played at it. Perhaps like Rilke and poetry before he encountered Cézanne. Why? Not because I wanted to write the Great American Play. I never saw myself as a second Arthur Miller, married to Marilyn Monroe reincarnated. Perhaps I'll reconsider that proposition.

I wanted to see if I could write a play. A simple question. And there was only one way to discover the answer. So my first play, like my first novel, began as a lark. Even more so. And it began with a coincidence. Like any good Alfred Hitchcock. Just because I was in the right place at the right time for something to happen. The right time in my life. I was at a production of Ibsen's *Hedda Gabler* at the University of Chicago. It was not a good production. My mind began to wander. That even happens to me during good productions of Ibsen. My fault, not his. So much else was going on. My second novel had been rejected. My marriage was falling apart. I tried my best to pay attention to Ibsen. To Norway. To Hedda. To the play itself. Hedda Gabler and the suicide of Eilert Løvborg. Especially his pivotal suicide.

How did we know that Eilert Løvborg really killed himself? That his death was due to suicide? My own question shocked me. So did my answer. We knew because the judge told us. Judge Brack. He was the messenger, the bearer of the bad tidings. He told Hedda and us that Eilert had killed himself. Was Judge Brack a reliable witness? Someone we should believe? A dispassionate observer? A messenger without a motive? Ibsen had given us a man to be respected. A judge. A figure of authority and respect. Ibsen set it up that way. But was this judge a man to be believed? An unprejudiced servant of the court? Was he to be believed?

Hell, no! Judge Brack wanted Løvborg dead. The two of them were rivals for Hedda's affection. Brack was actually pleased that Løvborg was dead, that he had "killed himself." His death left the judge, in Ibsen's words, as the only "cock on the walk." I wonder how many meanings that phrase conveyed in the original Norwegian.

So my question remained unanswered. Had Løvborg killed himself? Had it been a simple case of suicide? Or had he been murdered? If it was murder, the judge was certainly a suspect. And what better way to hide a murder than to call it a suicide? No murder. No suspects.

So I couldn't take Judge Brack's word at face value. He had a motive to kill Eilert. Did he have the opportunity? Good old Henrik Ibsen, crafty playwright that he was, had made sure of that. The murder, if I can call it that, took place between Act III and Act IV. So everyone had an opportunity. Starting with the judge. They were all off-stage.

And the judge was certainly not the only suspect. Far from it.

If Brack and Løvborg were competing for Hedda, where did that leave her husband, George Tesman? The play, as you remember, opens when Hedda and George Tesman are returning from their long honeymoon and moving into their house. So good ol' George Tesman had the oldest motive of all—jealousy. And opportunity. Just like the judge. It was intermission for them all.

Then there is Hedda's old friend, Thea Elvsted. She is Eilert's girlfriend. Eilert has been shacked up in the country with her before he comes to visit Hedda and George. No, this is not a soap opera. This is great literature. One of the pillars of modern drama. Ibsen all but created modern drama. Tragedies without class distinction. Not the tragedy of the Prince of Denmark, but of the newly married couple next door, just back from their honeymoon. No need to be a thane to qualify. Thea had the same motive and the same opportunity. So did her husband. She has a husband. She left him for Eilert. Now, there is someone with a motive. And he has more opportunity than anyone else. None of his time is accounted for, either during the intermissions or the acts themselves. Mister Thea Elvsted never even appears in Ibsen's version of the play. He would in mine.

And, of course, our heroine herself, our title character, Ms. Hedda Gabler, also had a motive. She may have been the first woman in modern literature to get married and retain her maiden name. Remember what happened to her. Eilert dumped her for Thea. Or so she thought. Then she married Tesman on the rebound. But her heart belonged to Eilert.

Those were my initial thoughts as I left the theater, following Hedda's suicide, off-stage again. Off-stage seems to be a dangerous place to be at the end of a play. Ophelia. Willy Loman. Hedda. Oedipus. Mrs. Oedipus.

But how to write it? And why?

The why was easy. I'm a writer. I construct situations that cause characters to interact. That's what writing is all about, putting characters into a plot. And that's what writing a play is about. Creating characters and giving them a situation to talk about, a reason to interact verbally. This was an opportunity I couldn't pass up. Think about it. Here I had a set of someone else's characters whose situation I could change. And whose actions, whose words would thus change. Old characters, great characters with new motives, new behaviors, and new words to fit the new situation. But I had to make it clear that they were both Ibsen's creatures and mine. How?

I'd throw in a touch of Pirandello. A bit of Wilder. Thornton, not Laura Ingalls. That may be a reflection of my age and my prejudices, but Thornton is the only Wilder I know. And I'd make it all very Brechtian. If not downright Stoppardish. I do know my theater. That allows me to borrow from the best. The hell with Polonius. Shakespeare borrowed from everybody. And it was the right time to do something different. My batting average was down to .500. My second novel had been rejected by more publishers than I knew existed. Time for a change. I'd write a play. But not a straight drama. Not the realism of Ibsen. Nor even of Arthur Miller. There goes the Marilyn Monroe fantasy. A piece of theater divorced from reality. A play within a play. Only more so.

So I set it as if a theater company, a semiprofessional one, in a city somewhere in the Midwest was rehearsing their final production of their "artistically acclaimed" season. Their play? *Hedda Gabler*. What else? This meant that each actor had two roles. One created by Ibsen, one by me. An example: The actor would not be cast as George Tesman, but as George Tesman as played by John Lindell, a pharmacist. That actor would be both Ibsen's Tesman and my Lindell, who was playing Tesman in the theater company's production of Ibsen's play. Got it? Actor X in the role of George Tesman as played by John Lindell. Lindell, by the way, played for the Yankees. He was both a pitcher and an outfielder. He wasn't too good as either.

Then I added characters. One was Dr. Stockman. He's from Ibsen's *An Enemy of the People*. In that play, Stockman becomes the enemy of the people, the medical scientist who fights for scientific truth and the good of humanity in the face of democratically manipulated self-interest. Why Stockman? I needed a figure with authority to examine the body and switch the cause of death. Murder, not suicide. The judge had misled us. Stockman has enough authority to overcome the judge's evidence. Even in Ibsen's own eyes. And adding Stockman gave me other opportunities, too. It allowed me to look at Ibsen in a broader context and to have Ibsen's characters react to both their own play and another play. And to allow me to show how interrelated all of Ibsen's plays are. And, of course, I added Thea's husband. And the producer and Ibsen himself. That's right, Ibsen. Good old Henrik, from author to subject. From playwright to character.

My play begins with Act Four of Ibsen's play and the announcement that Eilert is dead.

"Suicide," says the judge.

"Murder," says Dr. Stockman, coming up out of the theater.

And we're off. In comes Ibsen. Or Ibsen's ghost. Now comes the Pirandello bit. Are the characters Ibsen's? Or are they on their own once he has finished writing his play?

And it's not Eilert Løvborg who was killed. It was Burt Lenhardt, a young millionaire working through his inherited fortune by supporting this theater company's production of *Hedda Gabler* and, in turn, getting the role of Eilert Løvborg. Burt was, of course, having an affair with Margaret Lindell, John's wife. She plays Thea Elvsted. And also with Roberta Doerr, who plays Hedda and. . . . You get the idea, I'm sure. Art mimicking art.

It's sort of a murder mystery within a murder mystery or, better yet, a murder mystery mirrored by a murder mystery. Reality versus literature. Where does one begin and the other end? And vice versa. And can you always tell? With a lot about the limits of the latter. Or the former. And the process of structuring either successfully.

I wrote three versions. And the Chicago Theater Workshop, bless them, did staged readings of all three of them. They were in the right place at the right time. I was tired of writing by myself in a closed room. Or so I thought. I was on my own. I needed to be with people. A director. Actors. Other writers. What could be better?

That was three years ago. There have been no calls from Broadway. Not yet, at least.

Roger

The full text of the final version is available from the author on request. *The Gabler Affair,* a full-length play in two acts.

One Set [The same set can be used for *Hedda Gabler*].

Ten Characters: Seven actors, Three actresses.

September 10

Dear Rob,

You have asked a very good question, my friend. If I'm really so skeptical of Garcia and his results, or the selected pieces of his data that he has allowed the world to see, then why am I getting into the implant business? I could tell you what I sometimes tell myself, that I have no choice about it. The implantation story could be déjà vu revisited. The revenge of the neurosurgeons. Stereotactic surgery relived. That is a reality that I cannot sit by and idly watch play itself out. After all, we may have been this way once before, led down this same primrose path. By "we" I mean both American neurologists and our patients. We've been through all of this at least once before—starting before I was in the field. Neurosurgeons replete with testimonials and incomplete data had claimed that stereotactic surgery all but cured PD. And, believe me, that was how much of the hoopla and acclaim came about. Not from scientific vigor. And not from experts who knew Parkinson's disease.

According to the surgeons, all they had to do was destroy a small part of the brain, put a small hole in the right place, and they could reverse Parkinson's disease. No more tremor. No more rigidity. No more disease.

Where should the hole be put? How big should it be? No one knew for certain. They just knew it worked. It seemed so simple. All you had to do was put a small lesion in the brain and the PD went away. It was safe. And sure. And accurate. And effective. So damn effective. The tremor disappeared right there on the operating table. Right before your eyes. Any fool could see that.

Who needed neurologists? Not the neurosurgeons who did the surgery. And not PD patients. Until after the surgery. How long afterwards? A decade? Or even less? A year, a month, or a day. It makes a big difference.

This procedure was initially propagandized, a word I chose very carefully, by the late Irving Cooper. Am I being too judgmental? Too pejorative? Too unfair to the Messiah of stereotactic surgery? Stereotactic surgery was not invented by Cooper. He was one of the several neurosurgeons who helped develop the technique. He was not its Christopher Columbus. No matter what his fans may say. Let me tell you about a couple of patients of his. Two. Just two. The same number of cases published by Garcia. It's neither coincidence nor irony. It's just a number. More than one and less than three. One of Cooper's most famous patients was Margaret Bourke White. She was one of the world's best known news photographers. A superstar. A female superstar in a pretty much male world. Like a female driver driving in the Indy 500 and winning. She did a lot of work for *Life*. She was one of the great photographers of her age. She developed PD and her career was threatened by her progressive PD. Not just the tremor, but the slowness, the loss of agility. That was the real problem. Speed. She needed that speed. Without it she'd be lost. She went out on assignments all over the world and did all sorts of things to get her shots. She couldn't do that with PD. She needed a cure. Off to Irving Cooper. Could he help her?

What a question. Of course he could.

And save her career? Why answer the obvious?

So she underwent surgery. It was such a simple procedure. Safe, accurate, effective. Scientific progress. And she got her miracle. How do I know? I read all about it. They did a full picture story in *Life* on her and Cooper and her surgery. Her cure. Her miracle. No trip to Lourdes ever had better coverage or more fanfare. Patients read it. So did their physicians. If it cured a photographer of her tremor, it ought to cure everyone.

Patients flocked to Cooper. Doctors referred their patients to him. In droves. Neurosurgeons who knew nothing about PD started doing the Cooper procedure. You could now get your own miracle in your own neighborhood! No need to travel to New York. Or even a real medical center.

But what kind of a miracle was it? Lazarus revisited? Or merely a cured leper? Margaret Bourke White worked up to the day she went into the hospital, but following the surgery she never returned to work. Some miracle. White knew this. She had to. She was there. She was the one who used to work as a photographer. And Cooper had to know. He, too, was there. So did at least a few of her colleagues in the media. But not the public. Why not? Would it have made it harder to sell that issue of *Life*? Was it all for the sake of a story? She died a few years later from PD. That never made the cover of *Life*. Ain't freedom of the press wonderful? But I don't work for a newspaper. I need facts. So do my patients. And they deserve the facts, the truth. Maybe the readers of *Life* don't. But the readers of the *NEJM* do.

Hers is not the only story. I promised you two. This one is about a doctor. A doctor named Albright. You ought to recognize his name. Fuller Albright. He was one of the founding fathers of endocrinology. He almost started the field. He invented Albright's disease. He was even an editor of the *NEJM*. He, too, had PD. PD that was more severe than Margaret Bourke White's. More advanced. More debilitating. More in need of a miracle. He, too, went to Cooper for surgery on his PD and he ended up in a coma that lasted for years. A complication. A hemorrhage into the brain. I've looked and looked. I've searched the literature, but I can't find a record of this hemorrhage, this complication, this disaster, in any of Cooper's published data. Why not? Where had this piece of data gone? Don't ask me.

PD specialists know that the Cooper procedure had never been evaluated appropriately. When people finally started looking, the cures seemed to disappear, the complications appeared and those carefully placed lesions, the ones Cooper and other neurosurgeons put precisely where they wanted them, were all over the brain. All but random in location.

Why had that all gone on for so long? It's hard for me to be sure. I wasn't really there. I stepped right from my residency into the levodopa era. I became the miracle worker, the dispenser of manna. I guess in part it was due to our state of knowledge at that time. But in part it was the result of the Messianic tendency of several of the neurosurgeons involved. Including Cooper. For the short term, many of their patients improved and they were sure they had "cured" them. They had neither the interest nor the knowledge to carry out long-term follow-up studies and so they never did. Or were their motives far less innocent?

So the whole question of implants and whether they work is far too important for neurology to let this happen again. Neurology has grown up in the intervening years. There are good treatments for PD now and many centers for the study of PD. We can't let history repeat itself. There are ways to get the answers that are needed and the people to do it. So that's why I'm in the implant business. That's what I tell myself. I often believe it. Not always. And not completely. It may be the truth, but not the whole truth. Being a miracle worker is addicting. Need I say more?

The Committee on Human Investigation has already approved our implant program. It took them all of ten days. I'm still waiting to hear about the diet protocol—switching around all that protein. Less than ten grams of protein for lunch. That could be dangerous. We have to give that careful consideration. Very careful.

Yes, I knew that Muhammad Ali had flown to Mexico City and been seen by Garcia. And turned down the surgery. No, he is not my patient. And, no, he does not have PD. He is not really a candidate for an implant. There is no reason to believe it would help him. He has a more severe type of brain disorder caused by the frequent number of times his brain was injured. What happened to all those guys he beat up? They can't even afford to fly to Mexico City.

Roger

September 12

Dear Rob,

"The chase is on," to borrow a phrase directly from Sherlock Holmes. Or was it Watson? One of them said it. And "the game is afoot." I should remember which one. I dedicated my first book to him. Watson, that is. To John H. Watson, M.D., "whose modesty has prevented generations from appreciating what he taught Sherlock Holmes about the nature of diagnosis." How was that for putting my thesis right up-front? No hidden agendas. Subplot as subject. Did any of the reviewers even bother to read the dedication? It was there to tell everyone what the book was really about. Did reading it influence how they thought about the book? Not as far as I could tell.

Back to the real world. We have begun the search for a publisher who is willing to say "yes" and cough up some money to back up that positive response. My agent has picked out a publisher or, more correctly, an editor who works at a particular publishing house, an editor whom he thinks would be particularly in tune with this particular manuscript, and he has submitted *The Blind Observer* to that editor for consideration. The Rubicon has been crossed. Not in terms of publication, but in terms of my batting average. The denominator has now changed from seven to eight. It is now an official at bat. A statistic. I can never go back. Eight tries. Not seven. Let's hope the numerator also changes. And sooner, not later. I no longer have the heart for two years of resubmissions.

How did my agent pick which publisher? And which editor at that particular publisher? I have no clear idea. I don't even know which is more significant. The publisher, I think. My agent once told me about his process. Studying the lists of publications of each publishing house, meetings with various editors, discussions with other agents, inside information, trade news, gossip, rumor. He could try to do it by throwing darts at a list of all available publishers, like the editors of the *Wall Street Journal*. You must be familiar with that. They do it each year. In January the experts pick stocks to buy and the editors throw darts. At the end of the year they see which stocks did better. It's usually the darts. He doesn't do that, but it would probably work just as well as whatever he is doing. Maybe better.

Perhaps a Ouija board. No. They are more reliable than his track record has been. Notice that subtle change of pronouns from "my" record to "his." Just like Burt Shapiro. From "our" book to "mine." Ain't show business fun?

A sleep lab is one heck of a lot easier way to make a living. I don't make my living writing books. That's not what Chicago writers do. That's not our tradition. Nelson Algren may have said it best. He was the epitome of a Chicago writer. He wrote in Chicago, about Chicago, for the Chicagoan in all of us. Tough. Gritty. Honest. And painfully so. He wrote *The Man with the Golden Arm* and spent most of his life living in a third floor walk-up on the northwest side and not in an upscale neighborhood. Algren once heard that Harold Robbins was about to buy a casino in Monte Carlo. Robbins had received millions of dollars in advances while Algren was trying to find his bookie so he could collect the $17.60 his bookie owed him. $17.60. Real life in the big city. God never promised it would be fair.

There is now a prize each year for the best short story by a Chicago area writer, the Nelson Algren Award. The Robbins Award's for the best contract.

By the way, there is some guy in Cincinnati or Dayton who franchises sleep centers. That's right. Like McDonald's. Or Wendy's. Franchised sleep centers. Just what the world is waiting for. Who knows? Maybe the next time I'm in Indianapolis each of their malls will have its own sleep center. Between the Payless Shoes and West Coast Video. Right where the bookstore isn't.

Roger

September 16

Dear Rob,

Of course I'm writing a book. That's what we authors do. Especially when we have failed at being playwrights. We write books. Novels. Nonfiction. Collections. Crossbreeds. Books of every description. Diaries. Essays. Reference books. Memoirs. How else could all those publishers stay in business? To say nothing of all those editors and agents. Even letters. Collections of letters. Like Rilke's *Letters to a Young Poet*. Medawar's *Letters to a Young Scientist*. Or should it have really been the other way around? There's an interesting thought. Certainly they should be read that way. Rilke by young scientists and Medawar by young poets. That would do more good for Rilke's publisher than Medawar's. A real comment on our time.

I remember a lecture by Dylan Thomas. It was recorded. I heard that record when I was an undergraduate. I'm sure it's out on tape now or CD. In those few malls that do have bookstores. Even then I knew he was smashed. But that was part of the wonder of it. The poet stripped bare. With apologies to Marcel Duchamp. His mind at work. The mind of a poet. Churning over words. Ideas. Subjects. Rilke and the gold standard. W.C. Fields and his influence on the novels of Virginia Woolf.

Back to the letters. Our letters. My letters to you. Letters to a would-be writer. Letters to a physician who would be a writer. Letters to a fellow physician. Your suspicions are well founded. I am making a book out of our letters or, to put it precisely, out of my letters to you. It will become, when I'm done, an epistilatory novel. More out of Ring Lardner than Samuel Richardson, true, but either is a worthy sire. Does anyone still read Samuel Richardson? Does anyone still read Ring Lardner? I'm afraid to ask.

How can you be surprised? You remind me of a patient of mine. She begged and begged to be put on an experimental drug, to be part of an experiment, a protocol, to contribute something to our understanding of her disease, to be part of something bigger, to help every other patient with her disease. A noble sentiment, that. Distrust such sentiments. In their hearts of hearts that is not what most patients want.

I agreed. We signed her up. Informed consent and all and then she complained that we were studying her. But that's what scientists do, I told her. And writing books is what authors do.

And I am both a scientist and an author. Of sorts.

You do recall that I am an author, don't you? You must. That was why you wrote to me in the first place after all these years. Wasn't it? So I am putting together a book based on my letters to you. I am my own Boswell. What choice did I have? Potential Boswells have not been beating a path to my doorway. And I am your Boswell, too. But I'm not Pepys. This is not my diary. Not my journal. It is selective, not comprehensive. It is not supposed to contain all my thoughts and activities. God forbid. That would be too boring and too personal even for me. So of course it is filtered. Everything is filtered. Life is one big filtration process.

The book is not an autobiography. It is not the story of my life. So of necessity these letters are not about my life. They are about two of my lives, two of my professional lives, but my personal life is somewhere in between. And outside. Mostly outside. Your letter set the tone. Did you ask me about my life? My wife? Correction, ex-wife? My health? Two of our fellow interns have already died. Those were not your questions. So don't complain now.

Don't worry, my novel will consist of my letters only. Why? It's easier that way. I have complete control of the contents. The power of the author. The medical scientist can never achieve such control. No matter how detailed the protocol. The patient is always a variable beyond control. I've eliminated that variable. It's almost as good as publishing a book without having to deal with an author. The wet dream of every publisher.

And besides I have the copyright. Not you. Not the recipient, but me. The author. Trust me. It's true. I checked with Randy Jackson.

Do I know the ending? I never know the ending. My books are like one big research project. If I knew the ending, I wouldn't carry out the research. Even my mysteries. All I ever knew was that I didn't do it. But even that could change.

Roger

73

September 19

Dear Rob,

My lawyer talked to Burt Shapiro's lawyer today. My lawyer represents me, of course, and so he bills me for each and every minute of that conversation. Shapiro's lawyer represents Shapiro and he, too, is going to bill me. What a system. All in all, that discussion, at least as relayed to me, did not go very well at all. Burt is pissed at me. I guess that means there will be no more lunches looking down on Lake Michigan. I guess it also means that I will have to find another publisher for my next book of clinical essays. It is now tentatively titled *Son of Toscanini's Miscue*. More work for my agent. That's what he gets paid for. Or why he gets his percentage. I'll bet it also means I will have to go back to styrofoam cups of coffee in small cubicles without any view at all. Chicago has always been a tenuous place for writers. Ask Nelson Algren. He finally moved out of his third floor apartment and fled to New Jersey.

Shapiro's lawyer reminded my lawyer of the indemnification clause. Notice the shift from Burt to Shapiro. From friendly to formal. It would be easier to demonstrate this change in our relationship in French, moving easily from the informal to the formal, but I don't know French.

"What's that?" I asked him.

"That," he reminded me, "is the standard clause in which I, as author, indemnify the publisher against all libel suits."

"I didn't libel anyone," I protested.

"True, but you are involved in a libel suit."

"Touché." I am not entirely without any working knowledge of French. "So what's it mean?"

"They expect you to pay all of their expenses."

"All? Including all legal fees? I'm supposed to pay Shapiro's legal costs?" That's why I'm being billed for both ends of that telephone conversation. God forbid they make any conference calls.

"Yes. And his lawyers won't come cheap. I know them."

"Without having any control?" I inquired foolishly.

"Yes."

"That ought to be illegal."

"True, but we lawyers make the laws."

"Lawyers from big firms like theirs."

"Touché. I'll see what I can do." Then he added, "By the way, they are going to withhold all of your royalties."

"Withhold. . . ."

"For the indemnification."

"Don't tell me. It's in the contract."

"It always is," he advised me.

"No wonder authors hate publishers."

"Publishers also hate authors."

"I know, that's why they love publishing Conan Doyle and Dickens. Dead authors cause so much less trouble. And there's no one named Scrooge around to sue. I have to call my agent."

"Why?"

"To tell him that we'll need a new publisher for *Son of Toscanini's Miscue*."

"That's your new title?"

"It's better than *Toscanini's Miscue, Part II* or *Toscanini's Second Miscue* or *Toscanini's Miscue Returns*."

"True," he conceded.

"It's a good thing I have a day job," I said.

Randy didn't know what I meant. I wasn't sure I wanted to explain.

By the way, Bloom's winning percentage of .625 does not mean he was any good. I admit that his lifetime percentage was .625 and, of course, the average winning percentage is .500. For every win, there is a loss. Or, more properly, for every loss, there is a win. As any fan will tell you, a team is more likely to lose, to snatch defeat from the jaws of victory, than it is to win. And so it is with pitchers. The average average of wins is .500. But Bloom's .625 is statistically speaking no better than .500. He only had eight decisions.

Eight chances. Five wins. Three losses. Shift one and what do you get? Four wins. Four losses. .500. It's all a matter of statistical scatter. Ask any statistician you know. You must know one. Some of my best friends are statisticians. Look at the Parkinson Study Group. We do what we do because of statisticians. Ask any statistician. He can run any statistic he wants. Student's t. Chi square. ANOVA. Any statistical test there is. The answer is obvious. Five and three is not different from four and four.

Statistical scatter. The statistical scatter of a mediocre pitcher.

Then ask your statistician this. Your team has eleven pitchers. Four starters and seven also-rans. Seven mediocrities. If each of them is four and four, that's twenty-eight wins and twenty-eight losses. Good enough for fourth place. Let's throw in some scatter. Each of them is now five and three. Thirty-five wins. Twenty-one losses. Fourteen games above .500 and now you are fighting for the pennant.

Why? How did you get that good? Certainly not because the pitching staff is mediocre. They're great. Fourteen games above .500. I wouldn't trade them for any other staff in the league. Would you?

Take it from me, he was mediocre. Also meaning inferior, poor, second-rate. If you still like mediocrity, we have some pitchers we'd like to trade to you.

Roger

September 23

Dear Rob,

You sound like the boy who was amazed to discover that he had been speaking prose all of his life. Of course, learning how to practice medicine is little more than one long exercise in interpreting narratives. That ought to be obvious to all concerned. The tragedy is that not everyone understands that, neither the teachers of clinical medicine, the doctors whose lives revolve around that single skill, nor the students whose patients' lives will depend on that same skill. Nor even the subjects of the narratives themselves. "But I've already told the other doctors my story," they complain. "It's all in my records." As if records tell the real story. Any more than a box score accurately reflects what really happened in a baseball game. There's the old story about Shoeless Joe Jackson. Later it was told about Yogi Berra. Shoeless Joe complained to a sportswriter. The box score in the paper said he got one hit. He got two.

"A typographical error," the writer explained.

"Error, hell," Joe retorted. "The shortstop hardly touched the ball."

The point is that box scores never tell if it was a weak grounder that barely evaded the shortstop or a long line drive that whistled into deep left center field. Only historic narrative tells that. You had to be there and see it and then tell the tale.

So narrative is all and you understand that concept and employ it all day long as you navigate your way through a world of overlapping stories. That's all well and good. That's as it should be. That's what good medicine is all about. Not lab tests. Not sleep studies. Not fancy images on CAT scans or MRIs or even on ultrasound. Can you remember practicing OB without ultrasound? Another era. Ancient history. But those images are not what medicine is all about. Medicine is about narratives. *But*, and that is a big *but*, that doesn't guarantee that you will automatically be able to put together narratives in any other context or that whatever stories you reconstruct will have any literary merit. There are, Rob, two basic styles of medical histories that can be elicited even by those who understand the importance of such stories and these two very different sorts of tales are constructed by two separate types of narrators. Some physicians, like some people, see life as a series of events. Others see it as a series of ongoing stories, tales that are never-ending. To some, events happen and those events have a beginning and an end. They are final, complete unto themselves. To others, they are part of a longer narrative that never ends. There can always be another chapter and that chapter can change the reality of all of those chapters that came before. Which kind of tale do you construct from the events your patients bring to you? Is their vaginal discharge an event or a story? It is always part of a story. You know that. I know that. She knows that. But she may prefer to view it as an event. That's her choice. But do you make the same choice?

And, of course, the ending counts. At least to me. It doesn't let you reconstruct the rest. It merely changes it all. Like many a great piece of literature. You cannot reread *A Secret Agent* the same way once you know the ending. Or *Heart of Darkness*. Or even *Portnoy's Complaint*.

Once you know the diagnosis, you can no longer review the narrative in the same way. Hindsight is the greatest of all diagnostic tools.

And narratives change. Not only their substance, but also their structure and meaning. The narrative I construct out of events today is not the same one I would have constructed thirty years ago out of similar, if not identical, events and not just because I am no longer a halting medical student. I know more and I expect more. Not just more expectations but different ones.

Medicine is like Rome; it cannot be learned in one day, nor even in a long, consecutive stretch of identical days. It can only be learned as a sequence of long, complex phases. Phases that must be experienced sequentially, one phase at a time. In the proper order. And narrative plays a role in each of these phases and that role, what narrative means and how it is used, changes with each phase. It is only on looking back that I have understood these stages. On looking back and in observing others going through these same stages with varying degrees of success.

The first phase, the first use of narrative, is made up of the clerkships that we all take during the last two years of the standard medical school curriculum. It's there that narrative becomes the tool of learning. It is not part of biochemistry or anatomy. Or even physiology. Those subjects are compiled out of a myriad of events and facts. Cross-sectional facts. Science sans history. But then it all changes and history comes into its own. Not Thucydides. Not Toynbee. But each patient's own story, with you as the historian and the patient as the custodian of the source material. You learn to take a history. Starting with a CC (chief complaint), going on to HPI (history of present illness), and sailing on through social history, family history, education, employment, and environmental exposures, the entire ROS (review of systems), and then you put it all together into a coherent whole and go on to examine that whole. And what is learned in those two years? Did you ever ask yourself that question, Rob? I sure didn't until a hell of a lot later, when I tried to teach interns and residents, some of whom didn't seem to have learned what I had learned in medical school. That may well be a neurologist's approach. Defining what a particular part of the normal brain does in health by recognizing what the brain can no longer do when that part of the brain is injured.

What did they not know? Facts? Biochemistry? Anatomy? That was not it. They did not know how to recognize sickness. They did not know what sickness was. And health. Who was sick and who wasn't. How to recognize disease. How to convert history into disease. And where in the body that disease is located. What symptoms it's causing. How those symptoms relate to the disease itself. And all of these come out of the patient's own story, his or her narrative. A narrative used to define sickness with a capital S. To discover disease. Not just sickness as the absence of health, but disease as a positive force. And what makes up a disease? Any disease? And each disease? The Disease. That, of course, takes place within a patient, but in that stage of development each patient is primarily a case, a sick person possessing a disease. End of phase one.

And so begins the second phase, the internship. The year we spent together in the trenches of Presbyterian-St. Luke's Hospital learning grace under fire. It's no longer called an internship. It's PGY-1 now. Postgraduate year one. By any other name, it still retains its own aura. There is no time during that year to learn about *disease* in the same way that it should have been learned about in medical school. History is routine. It is extracted as easily as a small baby from a grand multiparous mother. As effortlessly. As automatically.

Who is sick? Who isn't? The presence of disease. All such questions must now be automatically answered. Sickness is not that easy to define.

Nor recognize. Nor quantify. And defining its limits may be even more difficult. In a way, it's the old uncle phenomenon. You see a man walking down the street, away from you; he's a block away. You recognize him immediately. He's your uncle. Are you certain? Yes. Why? How did you recognize him? That's not as easy to answer. How do parents know which identical twin is which? Don't worry. They know.

That's the process. That's what medical school was all about, but not everyone can recognize his uncle all the time. There are people who go up to strangers in error and are embarrassed. And they also walk right by their closest relatives without recognizing them. And the analogous thing can happen to bright people who will never make good doctors, not even good interns. That is one of the more peculiar, yet universally accepted parts of the process of medical training. Each phase must be successfully completed. Each skill must be obtained during its specific phase. One step at a time. Sure, those apt at learning can start getting the rudiments of stage two during stage one. And even stage three. Most do. That's all part of it. But you can't go back. If you haven't acquired the basic skills of clinical training during medical school, of the recognition phase of medical knowledge when you start phase two, forget it. With rare exceptions, you can't go back. There's no time in phase two, during a busy internship, to learn how to take a history, how to listen to a story, how to dissect a narrative and find a disease, any disease. The Disease. And more importantly, no one is willing or able to help you. It's assumed that you can do that. You already have your M.D. degree. Doctor of Medical History Taking.

So what is the internship all about? One thing and one thing only. Learning how to make decisions about sick people all by yourself at two o'clock in the morning. Grace under fire. Looking into the solitude of our soul and making decisions. And not just about one patient at a time. It's all about prioritizing and decision-making as an automatic skill. If Sherlock Holmes is really a physician in disguise, then there is little evidence that Holmes, or Watson for that matter, successfully completed his internship. Or that his audience is more sophisticated than your average third-year medical students. Holmes is brilliant at recognizing disease. He can sniff it out at its earliest stages. In its most unlikely forms. But can he make the right decision? In time to save the patient? Sometimes yes. Sometimes no. And only while working on one case at a time. What would he do if he had two cases at once? Three? Four? Or, like an intern, a full service? Ten, fifteen, twenty sick patients. At two in the morning. All by himself. With no Watson around to help pick up the pieces.

Clearly, if the intern has difficulty learning to recognize disease, to smell out sickness, to define illness, he or she will never learn grace under fire. You cannot make decisions about something you cannot recognize. If you have fallen behind during medical school, you now have a learning disability. One far worse than dyslexia. One that not only affects your life, but also kills other people. Sick people you didn't know were sick.

Stage three. You've survived the internship. So have most of your patients. On to the final phase. The residency. You can sniff out a disease. You can make a decision. What's left? Applying those skills to the organ system of your choice. If a resident has acquired the first two skills, I can teach him the third. If he hasn't, I can't. And he can't learn them. It's worse than dyslexia. It's a complete developmental arrest. Skills never learned cannot be honed. That's medical education.

Learning that the case history belongs to a particular patient, a patient with a life, with loves, triumphs, failures, frustrations, joys, stresses, strains, that is all extra. That cannot be taught. It's like learning to walk. It can be encouraged. It can be applauded. Rewarded. But not taught. The baby learns it all by itself. All babies learn to walk unless they have overwhelming neurologic problems. Deaf babies do. So do blind babies. But not all physicians learn that cases are patients, that patients are people. I have a patient. I've been treating her for years. She comes into my office to kvetch. One daughter was anorexic. We lived through that together. And a lot more.

Do I care about that daughter, whom I never met? You're damn right I do. That cannot be taught. And I have no idea what to do about that, Rob. No idea at all.

Roger

September 27

Dear Rob,

We did our first implant yesterday. And you thought that science moved slowly. Not this kind of science. Not the science of miracles. Did Our Lady have to wait for a Committee on Human Investigation?

Hell, no. She just appeared to Bernadette. And the rest is history. Lourdes to Werfel to Jennifer Jones. And people still flock to Lourdes. No one reads Franz Werfel. No one lusts after Jennifer Jones. But we still need miracles. Can miracles be reproduced? Can they be predicted? And if so, are they miracles?

Well, there have been no miracles yet, no new stars in the heavens. Wrong metaphor. But no complications either. At least no unexpected ones. Thank God. That was our biggest worry. You know medicine. It is Murphy's law on the loose. If something can go wrong, it does. Especially in surgery. Four neurologists are involved in the PD program here. Normally one of us makes rounds in the hospital each day. Not yesterday. All four of us were there pacing about expectantly. It was more like an OB waiting area than neurology rounds. Nothing we do is that dramatic.

What were we waiting for? Just for the implant to be completed. Not for a miracle. The patient won't get better for weeks or months. Just think how history would have changed if it had taken Lazarus a few weeks to rise from his grave. Would it still have been a miracle? Who would have been there to see it? To record it? To document it? Who would have bothered to wait that long? Only Beckett's characters wait every day, day after day, for an oft-delayed Godot.

Miracles either happen or they don't. Well, Godot did not arrive today. And we didn't expect him to. We have learned something.

Today all four of us went to see our patient in the ICU. "I want to read your second novel," the patient said to me. "The one about implants."

"After you're better," I said. If an implant patient wants to read *The Brain Implant*, why should I stop him? If we do enough implants and this trend continues, perhaps it could become a best-seller. But don't bet on it.

"I learned a lot about you in your first book," he continued.

"What did you learn?"

"About your taste in music."

We then went on to have a long, detailed discussion about classical music, ranging from Wagner and Von Bulow to Vivaldi and his all-girl orchestra including a certain bassoonist with whom Vivaldi was involved and for whom he wrote innumerable concerts. I'm sure they've been numbered. By Hoboken or whoever it was who numbered the works of Vivaldi. I just have no idea what the number is. She sure must have had a hell of an upper lip.

The patient's intellect and memory were obviously intact. His mind as sharp and keen as ever, which was great news. We'd been more than a little worried. After all, Frank Fain had gone through this man's frontal lobe. Things could happen, even in the best of hands.

"How do you feel?" I asked.

"My back is sore," he replied. "I kept her up all night." As he said that, he nodded toward one of my associates.

"Dr. Connors?" I asked.

"Yes."

"Was I here last night or was it a nurse?" she asked him.

"You were here. All night. You kept rolling me from side to side to relieve the pain."

And no matter what we said or how often or with how much conviction, we could not convince him that that was not true, that his doctor had not been at his bedside all night long. Physically he looked great. Awake. Alert. He moved all four extremities easily. He spoke quickly, loudly. Articulating well. He was in no pain.

"You look great," I concluded. "You'd think that all we'd done was operate on an ingrown toenail, not do a craniotomy and an adrenalectomy."

He looked at me quizzically. Then he looked toward the foot of his bed and lifted one foot and then the other. "An ingrown toenail." he said. "So that's why I'm in the hospital. I see."

I didn't. There were no bandages on his toes. I'm sure it's just temporary. Some swelling of his frontal lobe. No big deal.

Fred called again. He had heard that we'd done an implant. He wants us to operate on him. I told him we'd consider the possibility.

How had Fred already heard? I have no idea. We held no press conferences. We sent out no press releases. Only a few of our colleagues knew we were doing the procedure. And somehow Fred already knew. Ask him if you should buy Mylan.

Roger

September 30

Dear Rob,

Why did I know you'd start with *Amadeus*? Obviously it is easier to find than a copy of *The Assault* or even *The Third Man*. And far easier to locate than anything by Jacobsen. It's Jens Peter Jacobsen, by the way. His best works, according to Rilke, are *Six Stories* and a novel entitled *Niels Lyhne*.

Why did I suggest that you read *Amadeus*? A good question. You are not aspiring to become a playwright. And even if you were, I wouldn't have started you off with *Amadeus*. So I suggested it for none of the usual reasons. Not for structure. Nor movement. Nor character. Nor even language. A lot of plays do these things better.

But for sheer audacity. Triumphant audacity based on a unique conceit. The idea that Salieri killed Mozart did not originate with Peter Shaffer. The claim was made by Salieri himself on his deathbed, the ravings of a sick, demented, institutionalized old man. Alzheimer's disease before Alzheimer.

Writing a play about Mozart and Salieri, even about Salieri's killing Mozart, was also not an original idea. Pushkin, the greatest of all Russian poets, the great Pushkin wrote such a play one hundred and fifty years ago. And Rimski-Korsakov made it into a opera. Pushkin's short one-act play had many of the elements of the Shaffer play. Mozart's God-given genius. Salieri's jealousy. And Salieri's killing Mozart to preserve a place in the sun for all other composers. To make the world safe for second-rate geniuses like Salieri. It's one of the triumphs of CDs that people are recording everything. Even Salieri's operas. Even Rimski-Korsakov's *Mozart and Salieri*. I've heard it. I own it. On CD. You can get it at your local classical record store. Our newest anachronism. I wouldn't advise you to get it. It's boring. Most of his other operas are far better.

So what was Shaffer's triumph? What makes *Amadeus* not just successful, but deservingly so? He did something no other writer ever conceived of doing. He eliminated the writer in the story. He deleted da Ponte. Lorenzo da Ponte. Da Ponte was Mozart's librettist. He wrote the libretto for *Don Giovanni*, and *Cosi Fan Tutti*, and *The Marriage of Figaro*. The big three. The only three that have librettos that really work. Shaffer wrote him out of the play. There is no librettist. Mozart became his own librettist. The written words of his operas became his words, his conflicts, not someone else's words that he set to music. For a writer to see that artistic truth requires a skill, a degree of insight, a sense of detachment that is so rare that it borders on genius. Writers don't eliminate writers. They luxuriate in them. Shaffer eliminated da Ponte. And in so doing, he eliminated the ego of the writer. A lesson to be learned. Writers identify with all other writers. We write about them. About ourselves. See ourselves in them. Them in ourselves. The world is not a world of writers. A pity perhaps, but nonetheless true.

Rule one for a dramatist: Don't write a play about writing a play.

Rule two: As far as subjects, there are no other rules.

The same two rules apply to all other forms of writing. Of creativity.

It was an interesting thought of yours. I liked it. Dali as the first conceptual artist. A man before his time. It was the idea that counted, not the object. He had an idea of a suite of lithographs. That's all that was necessary. The actual lithographs merely documented his idea. And it is the idea that counts. The idea, not the manipulation of materials.

Message not medium. Orwell being out-Orwelled by Dali. But the only idea was to make money. And if it is the idea that counts, why buy a lithograph? Just think about it. There's no reason to buy one. You can't own an idea. All you have to do is to think about buying it. Conceptualize the concept. Once you've done that much, it's yours.

There's a notion Dali would never have bought. No way to make money.

You asked about paperback sales. So I'll tell you. Counting the sales of real books, the number of books sold by bookstores, is fairly straightforward. The bookstore orders the books. The books are sent to the store. Those that aren't sold are returned to the publisher and those that aren't returned are counted as sold. That's simple enough.

But that's not how it works for mass distribution of paperbacks. The ones that get into your local supermarket. They aren't even books. They're magazines. The manager of the supermarket doesn't order books. How the hell could he? What would he order? James Joyce? Ezra Pound? He has all he can do to keep up with his bananas. And kiwis.

So the magazine distributor does it all. And each week this distributor brings in the new magazines and the new paperbacks and takes out the old ones. And he determines how many racks of each book are displayed. Not my idea of free trade. And the unsold books are not sent back. The covers are torn off, tied into bundles, and those bundles of covers sent back to the publisher. Just the front covers. And these bundles are not even counted. Never. They are weighed. And that's how we know how many were returned. By weighing the front covers. The rest were sold.

That's why it is illegal to buy a paperback book without a cover. That book should have been destroyed. Its cover was returned as "unsold."

Aren't you glad you asked?

There is a new biography of Archibald MacLeish, one of the best second-rate American poets of the first two-thirds of this century. Sort of a poetic Salieri. Don't run out and buy it. Or his *Collected Poems,* or *J.B.*, his one commercial success, a play derived from Job. In the twenties, he was a lawyer. He'd graduated from Harvard Law School. That was his day job. He was offered a partnership. Instead he fled to Paris. To become a full-time writer.

Would you have done that? Is that degree of commitment within you? Would I? Don't ask!

Roger

October

Willie Sutton was a bank robber. His sole contribution to medicine was a quip that has become converted into a basic law. Willie never robbed anything but banks. The FBI, as well as the banks, took a dim view of such a penchant. As a result, Willie had been arrested and convicted several times, spending much of his life behind bars. When released from his last incarceration, he was interviewed by a newspaper reporter.

"Why," asked the reporter, "do you rob banks?"

"'Cause," Willie replied, "that's where the money is."

Harold L. Klawans
Newton's Madness

October 1

Dear Rob,

Who murdered Eilert? That was the sixty-four thousand dollar question. Do you recall when we were all that innocent? The world wasn't. We were. Life has changed. And not so much for the better. Is innocence still there to lose in quite the same way? Certainly not at the same age. Your question means that despite everything, despite your misgivings that I am not writing these letters to you personally but to some generic version of you, a second person plural generalized, you are still reading my letters. It's the curse of the reading class.

That means that I've succeeded. I've tweaked your curiosity. Isn't that what the writer of a mystery is supposed to do? You asked, so I will tell you. That, too, is one of the obligations of a mystery writer. The *who* must be revealed. At the ending. Nice and tidy. It's the writer's obligation. And I always meet my obligations. It's more the physician in me than the writer. More science than literature. Or art. No mysteries of Edwin Drood. No unfinished symphonies. We still read *Drood*. We look at unfinished Cézannes. And at Michelangelo's slaves only half out of their marble prisons. And listen to Schubert's *Unfinished*. And Mahler's *Tenth*. Bruckner's *Ninth*.

Does anyone study unfinished experiments? What a superfluous question. The beauty may be in the design, but the truth is in the data. Foreplay can only do so much. It has its limits.

So, I'll tell you. Ibsen, of course. Who else?

The murder took place off-stage. And Ibsen was off-stage with no stage directions or subsequent dialogue to control his actions. So Ibsen killed Lenhardt. Lenhardt, not Eilert Løvborg. He killed Don Lenhardt, the would-be actor who was playing the role of Eilert Løvborg. Why? Because Lenhardt was the worst actor he'd ever seen. Justifiable homicide if there ever was a case.

So now you don't have to see the play. As if you'd ever get the chance to. As if that one piece of stagecraft makes any difference. That's not what the play was all about.

My second play was shorter, less convoluted, less about itself, and far more dramatic. That play was entirely David's fault. He told me a story and then he charged me to do something with it. It was a story that had been told to David by a friend of his. It involved the friend's father. He told it to David because he had an obligation to tell the story. David told me the story and passed that obligation on to me.

Put simply, it was the story of an old man with all the problems of an old man. He was an old man with arthritis. Not merely a single attack of acute gout, bound to get better, but severe degenerative arthritis that was destined to get worse. He also had other problems, coronary artery disease, high blood pressure, what have you, and one more. One more key problem. This old man was a survivor of Auschwitz, a survivor whose body had been half destroyed during the Holocaust and who was receiving a disability pension from the German government. And therein was the story. Once every five years a physician would examine him to see if he still deserved his pension. *Still! If!* What a question. What a concept. What a proposition!

But that is not what gave the story its poignancy. The story had its own punch line. The man tried to describe his horrible, recurring nightmares. He tried to detail them to this examining physician, this objective evaluator, the man who would determine whether or not he was still disabled.

The doctor, the examiner, the determiner, his judge and jury, shook his head. This was not why he was there. Dreams didn't count. Not even nightmares. "We don't pay for dreams," the doctor said.

"We don't pay for dreams!"

Now there's a line for you. As great as any in the English language.

The story brought with it a charge, an obligation. Now I had the responsibility to act as a witness. For the story of the Holocaust did not end in 1945. For the survivors, that was the beginning of another phase that demanded both survival and suffering. But how could I best tell the story? With what details? In what form? He was not my patient. He had no neurologic history. I had only a snippet of his narrative. What more did I need? I am a writer. That's why David told me the story. And David is my best friend at the medical center, although that qualifying prepositional phase may well be superfluous and misleading. I had to use the story. I had to tell this story.

But how? By the construction of yet another clinical tale? From what elements? Could I do that? A clinical tale. Medical science for the layman. Or real literature. Or both. Or neither.

What they should pay for is an interesting question, neurologically. Such survivors have an increased risk of developing Alzheimer's disease forty years later. And Parkinson's disease. I've seen a number of survivors who developed Parkinson's. They all have one thing in common. They have all done very poorly.

Why? The worst side effects of our medicines for Parkinson's disease, the ones that prevent us from ever treating the disease effectively in the patient with that problem, are the psychiatric ones and these have three components: severe nightmares, progressing to hallucinations, and then to full-blown psychosis. Severe nightmares. Night terrors. Screaming out in the night. And that has happened to all of the survivors I've treated. Not a few. Not some. Not many. Not most. *All!*

"We don't pay for dreams."

Roger

October 4

Dear Rob,

Like every good Hitchcock screenplay, my involvement with Parkinson's disease began as the result of a coincidence. It was not the calculated result of a systematic survey of the "hot" areas of neurologic research. I carried out no such study, and even if I had I wouldn't have ended up in Parkinson's disease. It was a backwater, a dead end, or, in obstetrical terms, a cul-de-sac. Tay-Sachs was where the action was. So no survey. It was also not the result of working with mentors who had an interest in Parkinson's. Just the opposite. My teachers had an active disinterest in it. Coincidence. Sheer coincidence. Remember, Rob, a single coincidence at the beginning doesn't violate any of the rules of literature, either good literature or genre fiction. One per novel. And ever since then research on Parkinson's disease has been the dominant theme of my life as a neurologist. So has treating patients with Parkinson's disease. The two go hand in hand for me and always have. But it all got started by accident, a coincidence devoid of any irony.

My residency program in Chicago was supported by a grant from the National Institutes of Health. This meant that the federal government supplied money to pay my salary and also supplied sufficient funds to reimburse me for all expenses to attend one "educational" meeting each year. This was usually used to underwrite travel to the American

Academy of Neurology meeting. In the last year of my residency that meeting was held in Chicago, so I started looking for another meeting to attend. The only limitation was that the meeting had to be in either the United States or Canada. It was 1967. That was the year of Expo '67 in Montreal and during the first week in September Expo '67 featured two items of significance to me. The first of these was a visit from the English National Opera performing a number of modern operas, and the second was a meeting of the World Federation of Neurology Research Group on Movement Disorders. While I had no particular interest at that time in movement disorders, I did have a major interest in twentieth century opera, and the research group meeting at least held some promise. I was a young neurologist, looking for a research interest. That's not true. It held no promise at all. We are our teachers' prejudices. It did, however, fit the bill. It was a valid meeting.

I told my chairman that this was where I wanted to go. He smiled benignly and sent me on my merry way. While there, I saw Britten's *A Midsummer Night's Dream*, as well as his *Noye's Fludde*. I also managed to work in a Strauss opera and even a couple of sessions of the meeting. During one of these sessions, I saw George Cotzias present his initial result on the use of high doses of levodopa in the treatment of Parkinson's disease. His results were astounding. I recognized all the problems immediately. To illustrate his success, he showed movies of one of his patients before and after treatment. Now we show videos all the time at meetings, but in 1967 actual footage of patients was rarely shown. In the "before" movie, the audience saw a disheveled woman in a filthy hospital gown that was splattered with remnants of her last half dozen meals. Eggs here. Spaghetti sauce there. Or was it catsup? You get the idea. Her hair was unkempt, stringy, flaked with dandruff. She wore no makeup. She sat immobile, unable to get out of the chair. We next saw a movie of that same woman six weeks later. She had now been receiving levodopa for six weeks. And there she was, clothed in a new dress, her hair recently coiffured. Her lip gloss, rouge, and eyeliner had all been carefully applied. And now she was walking in the sunlight, in a lush green park with blooming flowers everywhere. Sure he'd loaded the dice. Cinematographically speaking. I was even smart enough to know that he'd also loaded the dice neurologically. In the two movies, she performed different tasks. Even though she was out of her chair "after" treatment and walking around, had she gotten out of her chair by herself? Could she have? Or had someone helped her? If someone had helped her get out of her chair "before" levodopa, could she have walked? Who knows? We never had the chance to see that. Even with these misgivings, the film was impressive. So were his data.

Then and there I decided that I wanted to study the use of levodopa in Parkinson's disease. I returned to Chicago and told my mentors that this was what I wanted to do. They thought that I was crazy. Cotzias was just like Barbeau and Birkmayer and the others in the field. They were nothing but charlatans and hucksters. They were not real scientists. They had never carried out proper scientific studies. They did clinical research. They were the mystery writers of medical science. Need I say more?

Garcia, in a way, reminds me of Cotzias. They both published in the *New England Journal of Medicine*. Enough said. I, too, have published there. More than once.

Roger

October 6

Dear Rob,

You probably never met Larry Solomon. I'm fairly certain that I did not know him back when we were interns together. I think that he and I first met after I had already finished my residency. He's head of dermatology at the University of Illinois. He's been chairman there for almost a couple of decades now. A long time. He's also the smartest dermatologist I ever knew. By far. He collects old books—mysteries. We were both guests of another Chicago area physician at a dinner party at his house last night. Over coffee and dessert, Larry told his Dylan Thomas story. The story took place in 1952. Larry was twenty-one. He was an undergraduate living at home and commuting to McGill University. He's from Montreal, of course. Knows Mordecai Richler and Leonard Cohen. He was a member of the McGill Literary Society. It was, he claimed, a fairly typical literary society, lots of girls . . . ah . . . women, a couple of guys who would later turn out to be gay, and Larry, who, because he was a native of Montreal and could borrow his father's car, became the official Literary Society gopher. And in February of 1952, his assignment was to go for Dylan Thomas.

Who, he wondered, was Dylan Thomas?

A great Welsh poet, he was told.

He'd never heard of him. In fact, he'd never heard of any Welsh poet as far as he knew, great or otherwise. But off he went to the airport to pick up the great Welsh poet.

"Why," I interrupted him, "if you'd never heard of Dylan Thomas, were you a member of the Literary Society?"

"All those girls," he reminded me.

He drove to the airport and picked up the great Welsh poet of whom he had never heard, Dylan Thomas. The poet was short, stocky, disheveled, yellow-looking. That was, Larry would later understand, a sign of Dylan's cirrhosis of the liver, his Laennec's cirrhosis, the end result of his years of excessive alcoholic intake. But Larry was still an undergraduate trying to impress the girls of the McGill Literary Society, not yet a medical student able to diagnosis jaundice due to alcoholic cirrhosis of the liver. But he could tell when someone was drunk. And Dylan Thomas was drunk. Already! It was four in the afternoon and the great Welsh poet was already under the influence, so to speak. "He was smashed," was the way Larry put it. Not very poetic, but direct enough.

"Take me to the hotel, my boy," Dylan slurred at him.

Larry hoped that some of what he'd heard was a Welsh brogue, not alcoholic slurring of the speech. Or did only the Irish have brogues? What did he know? He was just the gopher.

At the hotel, Thomas gave his shabby bag to the hotel porter along with a tip. The porter would put the bag in his room.

"Find me a pub, boy," Thomas ordered.

A pub? Larry thought for a moment. He knew the right one. It was right next to McGill. The college kids went there. It was owned by a guy named Andre. Andre's Pub. It was called Andre's shrine out of disrespect for the Catholic Shrine to St. Andre with all of its shed braces and crutches. Montreal's local version of Lourdes, without benefit of Franz Werfel. If I mention Werfel often enough, you may even read something by him. If you can find it.

In no time they were there and barely got inside before Thomas spoke out, "Get me some whiskey."

That was easy enough. They were inside a pub. So Larry, the gopher, ordered a bottle of Crown Royal. Rye whiskey for the great Welsh poet.

"Now, boy, I need women."

Women? Not woman? Women! Plural. Where? How? Larry had no idea. He was only an amateur gopher with no interest in becoming a professional. Is that what this great Welsh poet wanted? Professional women? Larry could not even get the word out.

"Women, my boy," Thomas bellowed.

Women!

Who would know where to get women? A professional gopher. A real gopher. A cabdriver ought to know. That's what everyone said. Larry went outside and hailed a cab. For ten dollars the cabdriver told him where to go for just what he wanted. And then the cabby drove Larry there—the local army barracks. Not the men's barracks. The women's.

Larry ran inside. He needed two women. They'd get all they wanted to drink for free. Two women. For one very drunk Welsh man. Free booze. Any volunteers? A car load. He picked two. One was built like a fireplug. Short, squat, tough. The other tall, blond, lanky, thin. Long blond legs. Dylan Thomas could take his pick if he could still stand up. That was his problem, not Larry's.

Back to the pub.

It was 6 P.M. The poetry reading was at 7:30. One and a half hours to go. One and a half hours of watching the great Welsh poet, the two women, and a succession of bottles of rye whiskey.

And watch he did. Until it was time to go. When it was, Larry went up to Thomas and told him it was time to go.

"Well, let us go now, boy," Thomas told him, drinking one more slug for "poetry."

Larry had to hold him up to get him to the car and then needed help to get him out of the car and backstage. Larry held Dylan up as they listened to all the preliminaries and introductions. Or rather Larry listened. Thomas was asleep on his feet. Snoring away. Even his snores seemed slurred. And this man had to read his poetry.

It was time. Larry jabbed Thomas. He startled into a form of consciousness. "Am I on, boy?"

"You are on."

Dylan Thomas strode to the podium. "Do not go gentle into that good night," he began. "Rage. Rage. . . ."

The voice was strong. Powerful. Mellifluous. There was no slurring at all. He went on poem after poem. Brilliant. Spellbinding. Greatness in real life. Real greatness.

The time was up. Thomas stepped back from the podium. Larry raced forward, just in time to catch him.

"Good show, lad," Thomas slurred. "Back to the pub, my boy."

Back to the pub it was. The women were still there, working on yet another bottle of rye.

"My flight," Thomas said as Larry eased him into a booth. Larry knew what he meant. He'd pick the great Welsh poet up in plenty of time to make his flight in the morning.

Larry got to the hotel early. He went up to Dylan Thomas's room, not knowing what to expect. The door was open. The women were gone, leaving a few obvious traces. Lipstick on a few cigarette butts. Not much else. No perfume. None that he could discern, for the room was filled with a stench, the stench of old vomit.

And there was Thomas. In bed, fully clothed, covered with his own half-dried vomit. Sleeping. Unarousable. Smashed beyond recall.

Larry had to do something. Thomas had to get on a plane. But what? He remembered the same movies from which he'd learned about women and cabdrivers. Thank God for "B" movies. Dylan Thomas needed a shower. A cold shower. Larry yanked and tugged and somehow managed to get Dylan Thomas into the tub and turned on the water. Warm at first. Then tepid. Then cold. As cold as possible. Which in Montreal in February is pretty darn cold.

It worked. Thomas awoke. The vomit began to wash away. "Good show, my boy," the great Welsh poet said. "It is time to leave this fair city."

Larry held him up and wrapped him in a blanket.

"To keep him warm?" someone asked.

"To protect my father's car," Larry responded.

He got Thomas into the car, to the airport, and into his plane.

And off to New York. For more readings. More pubs. More women. More cirrhosis. But few, if any, more poems.

Roger

October 7

Dear Rob,

Our first implant patient went home from the hospital today. The second one left the ICU and is now on the regular neurology floor. Meanwhile the third one came into the office for her last preoperative visit. Just part of the usual routine. Implants past, present, and future. We hope to get started on the protein diet protocol by the first of the year.

There have still been no miracles. No new stars have appeared in the firmament. Or in the field of neurology. Or neurosurgery. I wonder how many operations Garcia has completed by now? At least we have suffered no major complications. Knock on wood.

The first patient looks about like he did when he came into the hospital. No better. And no worse. His mentation is back to baseline. That took about a week. We still talk of Vivaldi. And Mozart. And Bach. He never mentions Salieri. What a fate for a composer. To exist only as a literary figure. As a character in a play. At least he's also a character in an opera, even if no one ever produces it.

Overall, patient number one's Parkinson's disease is unchanged. Number two is also unchanged, but we hadn't expected her to show any improvement yet. Even Garcia's miracles took more than a week.

I am sorry to hear that you have had absolutely no luck in finding a copy of Mulisch. I'll send you one. I have several for just that reason.

I'm sure David Garron must know who Jacobsen is and what he wrote and probably has even read all of his extant writings. How could you ask such a question? I once asked him if he knew much about Mandelstam, a Jewish Russian poet killed by Stalin. Weren't they all? He brought in five books of poems for me to read. Most of the individual poems were represented by at least two translations since no one translation could be perfect. So I'd get a better feel if I read both. And he also brought in three books of Mandelstam's prose. To get me started. Essays. Criticism. Started!

So you must understand if I have not yet asked him about Jacobsen. I have my reasons. I have not even started on all that Mandelstam. But I may ask him about Franz Xavier Kappus. He was the young poet who received all those letters from Rilke. He was *the* young poet. Two years after Rilke's death, Kappus published the letters. Under

German copyright law, I wonder who really owned those letters. Does it matter?

But let me remind you, my dear friend, you cannot publish my letters. The copyright belongs to me. And my heirs.

Roger

October 8

Dear Randy,

The letters between Tinker, the lawyer who is representing the not-so-late Martin Bloom, and Burt Shapiro's lawyer, the jerk named Evers, could be amusing. Tinker's assumption throughout seems to be that it was his Martin Bloom whose disease and death I described. Is his Martin Bloom dead? And buried? I didn't think you could libel a dead man. Or that a dead man could sue for libel. Or pay his lawyer's fees. His estate can do that. Thank God for that, there is still some justice in this world. Does Tinker represent his estate? According to the dates in my story, he's been dead for over a decade. Doesn't that mean the estate has been closed?

Hasn't the statute of limitations run out? I mean he's been dead for more than ten years. Or is it like murder? No statute of limitations. Capital libel, so to speak. And his claim that I used Martin Bloom's name for commercial advantage is beyond belief. It boggles my imagination.

What name? What advantage?

If I wanted a commercial advantage, I would have killed Mickey Mantle. Or Whitey Ford. Or had an epidemic that devastated the entire Yankee team from Andy Carey or Allie Reynolds to Yogi Berra. A to Y. No Z's. Zeke Zarilla played for us. So did Gus Zernial. Is death defamation? Is it libel? Are not the rumors of his death merely premature? If this isn't a frivolous lawsuit, what is it?

By the way, what does Marvelous Marty do for a living? What great commercial value has his name been to him? His brilliant career? All eighty-five innings of it?

Toscanini's estate had a better claim. I used his name because of its commercial value. No question about that. Toscanini is dead. So is my Martin Bloom. Even if Tinker's isn't. Nor Evers'.

Oh, well. Why should I complain? I shouldn't. Someday I'll put this entire story into a novel. Then the world will know my side of it. The writer's final revenge. And they can all sue me again.

Sincerely,

Roger Kramer, M.D.

cc: Rob

October 12

Dear Rob,

About suffering the old masters supposedly always got it right. Or at least Auden thought so. He wrote that they never got it wrong. Which is almost the same thing. You remember the poem *Musée des Beaux Arts*. Why the name of the museum? It wasn't the museum that mattered. It was the painting. *The Fall of Icarus* by Pieter Breughel the Elder. The one obvious problem with the poem is that without the painting in front of you it loses something. That got corrected the other day. I heard and saw Dannie Abse and his wife Joan give a reading/viewing of poems based on works of art. They projected a slide of the painting and one of them then read the poem. True parallel perception. Not trying to read and look at a picture at the same time. That can't be done. Which is why novels don't have illustrations. But true parallelism. Vision and sound. It's what our brains do best. And of course they stared at the Musée des Beaux Arts. It was wonderful.

But they got it all wrong. Not Dannie and Joan. The Greeks. And Breughel. And Auden. *His wings would never have melted.*

The Greeks had to have been able to figure that out. They knew the earth was round. The had even calculated its circumference quite accurately. By the way, no one ever believed that the world was flat—no one who was at all educated. The Romans knew the earth was a globe. So did educated Europeans ever since. The argument that Columbus had was about the circumference and he had it all wrong. He thought that the Indies were only a couple of thousand miles to the west. So he traveled those couple of thousand miles and thought he had reached the Indies. His calculations were off. But no one had thought the earth was flat and the ancient Greeks had been right all along. The earth was a globe.

And as you climbed up a mountain, it got colder. The higher you got, the colder it got. And the sun was so damn far away. Icarus could never have gotten close enough to have gotten warm enough for his wings to have melted. No melting, no hubris. No moral. If God had wanted man to fly, he would have given him airline tickets.

About suffering they were not wrong. The world little noted nor long remembered what happened to that poor kid whose wings melted. Icarus was falling into the sea. The ploughman plowed on, the ship sailed calmly on its way. Life went on. Who even noticed that the trains chock full of people only went into Auschwitz? Never out. Just in. Day after day after day after day. Month after month. Year after. . . .

Breughel got something else right. Meige's disease. It's a movement disorder. Named after the French neurologist who first described it around the turn of the century. Henri Meige. It consists of prolonged forceful closure of the eyes and spasm of the lower face. But Breughel saw it first. Three hundred years earlier. He painted an old lady with forced eye closure and facial spasms into one of his great genre scenes. She, too, would have paid no attention to Icarus. She would have had an excuse. Her eyes were closed. What was everyone else's excuse?

Spell-check did it again. Why is ploughman ploughman? And plow plow? And not vice versa? Or merely random? Genug.

Roger

October 16

Dear Rob,

Of all the reviews, why did your mother send you that one? The *New York Times* loved that book. The *Chicago Trib* liked it a lot. The reviewer for the *San Francisco Chronicle*, a lawyer, raved about it. And the *Sun Times* reviewer trashed it. And that's the one she sends you. Why? I know why; she lives in Chicago and reads the *Sun Times*. Why she reads that rag I'll never know.

Certainly the reviewer does have every right not to like *The Expert Witness*. Hell, there are parts of it that I don't like anymore and doubt that I ever really did. Fewer than in some of my other books, but still a reality. He also has every right to explain why he dislikes the book. He has every right not to like my style of writing. Too clipped for him. Too staccato. His word, not mine. Too jarring. That's his right. That's what makes horse racing and literature and, my God, read what he wrote, if he's even partly on the right track, I may have succeeded. All of my hard work may have paid off. I have a writing style. A style all my own. I say what I want to say in the style I want to use. Isn't that what differentiates writing from typing—style, whether leisurely, langsam, or staccato. I'm not sure langsam is the right word. It's German and staccato is Italian. Isn't that like mixing metaphors? Would it be adagio assai? That's the directions for the funeral march in *Eroica*. I'll stick with langsam. A style, Rob. And it must work. Even Hines admits that I have the ability to make arcane medical details understandable to laymen. So my style must not be all bad. But this William Hines, who is identified as a writer on scientific and medical matters, wrote some things that no barely competent first-year medical student would write. And that he has no right to do. None whatsoever. And what recourse do I have?

One of my chapters was about a woman who fell and broke her hip. I, as a neurologist, rhetorically ask why she fell. Beware of rhetorical questions. They fall somewhere below coincidences. Fell, not tripped, as he suggested. The difference between tripping and falling is usually a simple matter of asking the patient what happened. History Taking 101.

"What happened?"

"I fell down."

"Did you trip?"

"No."

Neither was she hit by a car. Unless that car was somehow speeding through her living room.

So I played neurologist. I often teach medical students what it is that differentiates a neurologist from every other doctor in the world. It's this patient. A patient who falls and breaks his or her hip. That mobilizes everyone. The ambulance, the paramedics, the ER physician, the radiologists, the anesthesiologist, the orthopedic surgeon, the internist—to prevent post-op complications. All good. All right. But no one asked why the patient fell. That's what neurologists do.

Why did the patient fall? Spontaneous falls happen for one of two reasons. Reason one: fainting. Is that staccato enough? But what is fainting? Why do people faint? They faint when the brain doesn't get enough blood. A cardiac problem or low blood pressure.

Reason two: Parallel staccato structure. Some part of the brain isn't working right.

But what does Hines write? "An even more frequent reason for falls in old women is osteoporosis." Any idiot knows that. Any damn fool but this hotshot neurologist. Well, he's the damn fool. Osteoporosis does not cause falling. Not ever! In legal parlance, it is not a competent cause of falling. It makes it more likely for a fall to result in a broken bone but it doesn't cause the goddamn fall.

But there it is. He's written it. He's attacked my competence as a neurologist. On what basis? What medical school did he go to? How many people travel from hell and go to ask his diagnostic help to figure out why they fell and broke a hip? They know it wasn't osteoporosis. Only a damn fool would make that diagnosis. But I am helpless. There's nothing I can do. The system allows no response.

Then he adds insult to injury by defending Ezra Pound. One of the tales in the book is about Pound and how his psychiatrists had prevented him from being tried for treason. He'd been in Italy during the war and had made propaganda broadcasts for Mussolini, broadcasts filled with anti-Semitic and anti-American sentiments, urging U.S. soldiers not to fight. Anti-Semitism, Hines tells me, is no crime even though it may be tacky! *May be tacky!* Tacky is his exact word. Who the hell does he think he is? Is anti-Semitism like eating soup with the wrong spoon? Or with your elbow on the table? Or perhaps like preferring Madonna to Ella Fitzgerald? Just a bit tacky. And his editor let him print that. Anti-Semitism *may be tacky*. Not *is,* just *may be*. What about hating blacks? Is that just a social indiscretion?

And if making propaganda broadcasts for the fascists is not treason, then I don't understand the English language. Look up treason in your dictionary. Or in the Constitution. It is defined there. Has Hines ever read that definition? Giving aid or comfort to the enemy. That's it.

But anti-Semitism is more than tacky. His review is tacky. Shabby. Cheap. What Pound did and what his psychiatrists did to protect him was not tacky. It was not a social indiscretion.

Burn that damn review.

Roger

By the way the dictionary on my word processor didn't accept "Eroica." Wanted to change it to "Erotica." Beethoven would have loved that.

October 21

Dear Rob,

Your fax came on the heels of a fax from the Parkinson Study Group. Theirs was another in a series of urgent missives. Emergency epistles. People seem to believe that since faxing a letter assures instantaneous transmission, the answer should also appear instantaneously. As a reflex. The 1990's version of simultaneity. No time for consideration. No foreplay. Just plunge ahead and respond. I am answering yours first.

The PSG has been concerned about conflicts of interest. Not just overt conflicts but also the appearance of any such conflict.

What do I mean by overt conflict? That's easy. The PSG knew all about the results of DATATOP a year before they were finally published in the *New England Journal of Medicine*. One whole year. When we first learned about it, Mylan was selling, if memory serves me correctly, for about $3 a share. I think it is now somewhere between $20 and $25. That's not a bad increase. Let's assume it is now $24. That is a seven-fold profit on your investment in a year. Thirty thousand dollars would have become damn near a quarter of a million. But it would have been a conflict of interest for any of us to invest. It would have, in a sense, been insider trading. Although I am not sure that any of the present laws or regulations would consider it such. After all, we are all individual investigators. We are not employees of the drug company. We are scientists. We carried out an experiment. We got the results of that experiment. Is that insider information? Is it really a conflict of interest to act upon that which we believe is the truth? Since, however, we are continuing to study the drug, we all agreed that it would be totally inappropriate for any of us to either act upon the information in our possession or divulge that information to anyone. Needless to say, within a few weeks of our secret meeting, during which we all learned the results, Mylan stock began to increase in price. So much for secrecy. Who leaked the information? Who learned it? I'll bet Fred Gould did. How? I'll never know.

There is another issue of conflict of interest that we are now debating. Should we give lectures that are sponsored by any company whose drug we are studying? This is such a complicated issue. Should we give lectures sponsored at all by drug companies? If those of us who are experts on Parkinson's disease all refused to do that, who the hell would give the lectures? Someone asked me a key question at the end of my lecture in Indianapolis. They said that I had relayed to them some fairly interesting information about a drug distributed by Sandoz. It was true that I had. But why should they believe me? After all, wasn't my lecture being sponsored by Sandoz?

A very good question. I pondered it for a moment. I then looked the questioner straight in the eye and responded, "You are right to be skeptical. After all, I am human and every man probably has his price. I, too, have my price. Unfortunately for me, Sandoz is too cheap to meet it. I give the same lecture no matter who supports me."

David stopped by my office this morning. Poor David. He is hobbling again. His gout has recurred. It got better for a while as he observed the natural history of his disease. And now he is worse again. I may have to buy him a gout stool.

This time he's on medication. Indocin. So much for the natural history of disease. Observation has its limits. And David is back in the fold. A true believer. No longer a heretic. His Albigensian heresy has been crushed. Without a formal crusade. Merely a recurrence of pain. Pain and suffering. And the institution of treatment. Therapy. Medical intervention. Doctors at work. And so all of his friends are his friends again. All those physicians he's known for decades.

They are smiling. Triumphant. Victorious. Vindicated. They rejoice. Why? Because David is in pain. Ain't medicine wonderful!

Roger

October 25

Dear Rob,

Spare me all editors. No, not all editors. Not the real editors who have been through it all, but all the others. Why do they do the things that they do? I have no idea. I suppose they must. The ideal world for an author would be to publish a book without having to have a publisher, an editor, or a vice president of marketing. Just a manuscript, a printing press, and bookstores with shelves lined with his or her book and lots of customers clamoring to buy that book. My book. Now that's the stuff dreams are made of. Always borrow from the best. Hammett knew that. That's the fantasy.

The sentence as I had written it was simple and straight—concise. Three words. Nothing out of Victor Hugo. Or Faulkner. Hemingway could have written it. Or any reasonably educated seventh grader. "I was dumbfounded."

Simple enough. Anyone could also understand it. Even that same reasonably educated seventh grader. It communicated how I felt—"dumbfounded." Short. Staccato. Clipped. My style. The style Hines hated, but my style. That sentence used to be in an article I had written for *Discover*. The project itself was a fairly interesting one. I was converting science into literature, or perhaps medicine into writing. Or an admixture of both. It was the story of a patient of mine. For the purposes of literature, I had renamed her Roberta Rose Richards. Three R's. Her original name had had the same alliterative quality, but with a different sound. I'll never tell which one.

She had come to me because of her Parkinson's disease, which no one else had been able to help. I treated her for the next decade and I, too, never helped her, despite all my machinations. But I did something her other doctors had not been able to do. With a flurry of scientific bravura, I had proven that she did not actually have plain, old-fashioned, garden variety Parkinson's disease, but a Parkinson disease-like state that would not respond to any of the medications within our arsenal because she did not really have Parkinson's disease. Unlike the others, I now knew what she had. I'd obtained gnosis. I'd replaced ignorance with knowledge. And in doing so I'd made scientific progress.

And in a way she became famous. I published her full story in *Neurology*. No rejection slips. One submission—one acceptance. Life was like that in those days. I was on a roll. And none of it ever helped her one bit. Science had advanced and that advance had not helped Roberta Rose Richards one iota or one scintilla. Or one anything else. Such is science. Such is progress. And all she ever wanted was to get better.

That was the story I wrote for *Discover*. I called it, "Such Is Fame." They called it "Fame and Misfortune." My story emphasized the difference between my goals and Roberta's. My triumph and her fate. My failure. The editors there loved the irony. They love irony more than most first-year college English instructors. I know that's hard to imagine, but trust me on this one. Their edited version of my story emphasized the role Roberta's suffering played in increasing our understanding of the brain. Ah, the irony of it all.

In my story, "I was dumbfounded." In their edited version, "I was flummoxed."

Flummoxed! I wasn't even certain I knew what that verb really meant. I turned to my dictionaries. It was there. Its origin was unknown, just like the origin of Parkinson's disease. But its meaning was known, at least to the editors of the dictionaries. "Bewildered. Disconnected. Baffled."

I now knew what it meant. It meant dumbfounded.

The dictionary added one more phrase, a qualifying phrase. "Slang. Chiefly British slang."

For the second time in my entire life I fully understood a comment that had been made by the great British conductor Sir Thomas Beecham. Beecham, it seems, had hated all recording engineers. These men had transformed his essentially ephemeral art into permanent contributions to world culture. Why did he hate them?

"I have spent my lifetime," Beecham said, "controlling the horns in Beethoven's *Eroica,* a lifetime striving for the balance I know is there and with one flick of the wrist, any damn fool recording engineer, a fool who has all he can do to carry a tune, can destroy that balance."

Beecham, too, had been flummoxed, but he had the right of final rejection. He could refuse to allow the record to be released.

So did I.

And I exercised my right. Once again I became dumbfounded. Flummoxed became superseded. Obsolete. Past history. Old British slang. The first time? That had been in a chapter I had written for a textbook on the chemistry of the brain in neurologic diseases. Not destined for any of your best-seller lists. My chapter was to be on Parkinson's disease and related disorders. What else? I opened the chapter with a simple sentence in which I wrote that the observation that levodopa improved the signs and symptoms of Parkinson's disease suggested a relationship between the chemical dopamine and Parkinson's disease. Simple. Straightforward. Maybe not Hemingway, but certainly not Faulkner. And never Victor Hugo.

"Suggested," I had written. "Posited" came back to me. There it was right in the middle of my opening sentence, right in the middle of an opening sentence that had replaced mine. Displaced mine. Dislodged mine. Superseded. Supplanted.

Was this the right chapter?

I checked the title. It was.

Had I written it?

I checked the byline. I had.

But I hadn't. Not this. I was, to coin a phrase, flummoxed.

I reread the cover letter. These were the editorial proofs. I had forty-eight hours to check them and then they would be printed. Forty-eight hours! Forty-eight hours and I couldn't even get by the first sentence. The first verb. Posited? Posits. To posit.

What the hell did that mean? A posit was something a dog left on the middle of the carpet. It was also a verb, I soon learned. An archaic verb.

Other new words appeared throughout the chapter in the place of old tried and true friends: Antipodes. Contretemps. Irrefragable.

The list went on. I didn't. The editor of the book was a friend of mine. His wife had been an English major. Old English, I assumed. Ye Olde English.

What to do?

I gave my friend three choices. He could publish the chapter as I had written it. He could publish the chapter as rewritten, but under the byline of the editor who had done the rewriting. Or he could go to press without the chapter. And I really didn't care which he did, but this version could not be published under my name. That was in 1971, four years before I wrote my first novel, but I already knew that I was a writer and no editor could make me say what I wanted to say in any way that I didn't want to say it. No posits. No antipodes. And nothing that was irrefragable. I never even looked that one up.

I forgot to answer your question. What a question! Carbons? Do I keep carbon copies? Or Xeroxes?

Get serious, Rob, this is 1992. I have the originals in my PC. Not just the drafts you received, but further revisions.

I know that the letter writer retains the copyright because I asked my lawyer, the one who is doing battle with Martin Bloom. I got a letter from Erich Leinsdorf, the great conductor, and wondered who owns the copyright. Apparently Leinsdorf does. The words but not what he told me. He had been on call for Toscanini's last broadcast in case The Maestro got ill and could not go on. That's the broadcast I analyzed in *Toscanini's Miscue*. It was Toscanini's Miscue.

Read the book.

Roger

This time it accepted "Eroica." Ain't progress great?

October 30

Dear Rob,

STRIKE ONE!

You guessed it. *The Blind Observer* was not picked up by the first publisher. They turned it down flat. They made no offer at all. They don't think that a mystery about AIDS will sell. I feel like *Casey at the Bat*. I'm just standing here with my bat on my shoulder. Somebody is pitching. My agent. Someone is catching. And someone else is calling the pitches. And after all of them get finished doing whatever it is they are doing, I'm the one who could strike out. What exactly do agents do?

Don't ask me. I don't tell my agent how to practice agenting and he doesn't tell me how to practice neurology. He's one of the few people who doesn't. My patients certainly do. And their husbands and wives. And their children. Not the ones who come in regularly with their sick parents. Never them. They know what I'm doing and how I do it. It's the ones from out of town who haven't seen their fathers in a decade or more. They come in. My God, Dad is sick. Hell, he's been sick for the last ten years. When they left town he was fine. It must be that doctor. We've got to get him to help Dad. I've been down that road too damn many times.

My agent seemed surprised when I talked to him, but was he really? Is that what caught him off guard? Their rejection of a book of mine? That's not surprising. It's happened so often that it's routine. Like a called strike during a prolonged hitting slump. I'm no Ty Cobb. People throw strikes by me all the time. Or was it the reason for their rejection that tripped him up? Or was it the fact that the mystery involves AIDS? That *The Blind Observer* is really about AIDS. All you were afraid to know and therefore never dared to ask. Sugarcoated as fiction.

I wish I actually knew. Did he read it or merely write a cover letter and send them off together? Or did he know what it was all about and think that AIDS would sell? The editor who rejected it sure as heck didn't.

Strike one. But here I am, back in the batter's box, ready to take another swing. It has been one of those weeks. One damn thing after another. The *New England Journal* also rejected an article of mine. And it wasn't even about AIDS. All was not a loss. *Neurology* accepted a paper, as did *World Neurology*. That one had already been rejected by *Neurology* and *Archives of Neurology* and *Annals of Neurology* and *Brain* and . . . a couple of other journals, the names of which I've already forgotten. Thank God no one keeps track of such things. In science I still am batting 1.000, just like everybody else. Ain't science great?

Roger

October 31

Dear Rob,

It's become a routine. We're almost cranking out a brain implant a week. It's 11:15. None of us are pacing the hallways. We only did that for the first patient and the second patient. Now we just sit around and wait. No longer the anxious husband. More like the waiting grandparents. Waiting for a call from the intensive care unit. Or from the OR.

The implant started at 7:30 and sometime later this morning or early this afternoon the surgeons will be done and the patient will be transferred from the OR to the ICU and we'll go over to see him. No mad rush. Just another set of rounds in the ICU. Another routine miracle. Bernadette at work. Was it routine for her? I'll have to read my Franz Werfel. I never read it. I only saw the movie. Don't tell anyone. I'll deny it. The phone is ringing. Time to go.

I'm back. It's 2:00 P.M. They finished the operation at 11:45 and after (but not before) our noon lab meeting, we all walked over to the ICU.

The patient was awake and alert. And in little, if any, pain. He responded to our questions rapidly and cogently. He didn't want to read any of my books, but no one else thought he was confused. That was a first.

There have been no miracles yet. The first couple of patients may be starting to feel better. Less tremor. Less slowness. More energy. Better balance. Improvement. The road to success? Perhaps.

I talked to Fred again. I finally told him that he is not a candidate for our program.

Why not?

He lives too far away for constant evaluation.

Perhaps he could try New York, I suggested.

"Or Mexico City," he countered.

Or wait until the results were clearer, I added, knowing that that was not really an alternative for him.

Waiting is not what he does best. By the way, he did buy Mylan at three. And sold it at eighteen. He's not a glutton. How many shares? Over twenty thousand.

"How," I asked, "did you know?"

He hung up.

Roger

November

Who the heck was the shortstop for the '27 Yanks? What kind of a question was that for a forty-four-year-old neurologist to worry about? Paul Richardson knew that he ought to be thinking about more serious matters: the research lab, the paper he had to present in New York in less than a week. The forty minutes or so he spent each morning driving from Highland Park to the hospital were too important to waste.

It was Gehrig at first; Lazzeri at second; Jumping Joe Dugan at third; Irish Bob Meusel, Earl Combs, and the Babe in the outfield; with Pat Collins, Johnny Grabowski, and Benny Bengough behind the plate. So many people got that wrong and said Bill Dickey, but Dickey didn't get to the majors until '28 and didn't become their regular catcher until '29.

But who the hell played shortstop?

Harold L. Klawans
Sins of Commission

November 1

Dear Rob,

Good writing may depend, more than anything else, on tenacity, on the tenacious pursuit of an idea to its ultimate conclusion. That idea can be a character, a plot, a scene, an emotion. Even a single line. "We don't pay for dreams." Or, better yet, "The stuff that dreams are made of." Or "Exterminate the brutes." Or "Mr. Kurtz, he's dead." That's two for one. Whatever you start with, it's the tenacity with which it is pursued that makes the difference. And that tenacity can be applied intensely or leisurely. And, yes, that makes writing pretty much the same as science. I'm not talking about genius here. Not about those few who have the ability to see things differently than the rest of us. To be Wittgenstein and see a problem from a different perspective. But without tenacity what good is genius?

David Garron came by today. After weeks of searching he had found what he was pursuing. David is tenacity incarnate. That's what got me off on this tangent. He is tenacious whether his quest is medical or scientific or literary. He has the same tenacity, the same intensity, in both worlds, and that is a rarity. Most people just dabble in their avocations. Others become their avocations, and their supposedly true vocations assume second place. All too often a distant second. Not so with David. He brings the same passionate curiosity to his patients that he brings to his poets and his other literary pursuits.

I am no longer like that. I was once. When I was writing a review article on some scientific subject, I was as tenacious as tenacious could be. I dug out every reference. No matter how old. Or how obscure. Or in what language. As long as it was in English, German, or French. No longer. I have not got the patience for that any more. I just can't do it. Was it all veneer? My reputed scholarship. Surface, not substance? A game I played at. Or after twenty-some years refining the same substances, I have just become bored. So literature to me is what cocaine was to Sherlock Holmes. If only life were that simple.

The object of his quest was Alma Mahler, the wife, lover, mistress, muse, all of the above, of such luminaries as Gustav Mahler, Walter Gropius, one of the founders of the Bauhaus and one of the best architects of the twentieth century, the greatest of the German-speaking world, Gerhart Hauptmann, the great Viennese expressionist playwright, the painter Oscar Kokoschka, and the novelist, Franz Werfel. Back to him again.

What a lineup, Rob. Like the '27 Yankees—a string of Hall of Famers if there ever was one. And all fascinated and dominated by the same woman, sequentially, simultaneously, what have you. It would be as if Marilyn Monroe had gone from Arthur Miller to Marc Chagall to Saul Bellow to . . . anyone but the Kennedy boys. Forgive me, Joe DiMaggio, but that is a lineup in which you just don't fit. The all-time Yankee all-star team, yes, but baseball is only baseball. Diversion. Passion. Metaphor.

And what is my image of her? Alma, to me, is the eternal *femme fatale*. Marlene Dietrich with a Ph.D. in European intellectual history from the University of Chicago—or rather from the University of Vienna. That's my vision of her, eternal beauty, eternal youth, eternal sexuality. One part Marlene Dietrich. One part Sophia Loren. One part Ingrid Bergman with a generous helping of Simone de Beauvoir. Or at least Lillian Hellman. Or Marguerite Duras. Circe, at the very least.

And David had found a picture of her. Where? In a biography of her last husband, Franz Werfel, author of *Song of Bernadette*. The movie version starred a very young Jennifer Jones. Alma was undoubtedly too old by then. He also wrote what remains the best known piece to come out of the Armenian Holocaust, *The Forty Days of Musa Dagh*.

My fingers shook as I took the book from him. I would finally actually get to see her. Marilyn Monroe. Sophia Loren. Ingrid, Gina. My grandmother! There she was. Tall, heavy, broad-shouldered, broad-beamed, long-faced. Looking just like my grandmother, only more so. My image was shattered. Gone. It had not been her beauty that had turned them all on.

Her marriage to Mahler had not been a happy one. By 1910 he was composing his Eighth Symphony while she was shacked up in a hotel with Kokoschka. And Mahler knew all about their affair.

What could he do?

See Sigmund Freud. What else? This was Vienna, after all. And what a Vienna. So the pivotal symphonist of the turn of the century went to see the Father of Psychoanalysis to be analyzed. Not a complete analysis. Not four times a week for a lifetime. Mahler didn't have that kind of time. Or patience. Nor did Freud. So they met for a brief consultation. A one session analysis. Those two geniuses spent four hours together one afternoon somewhere in the Netherlands, where Freud was on vacation and where no one else could observe that they had even met.

Some analysis that was. Freud never let these time constraints stand in his way. It might not be sufficient to gather all of the needed data but it was plenty of time for him to draw all of the necessary conclusions. More out of Alice than Anna O. Wonderland revisited. Sentencing first.

Freud reached his verdict. First for Alma. She had been seeking a father figure. Remember, this was based on four hours wandering in the woods with Gustav. So Alma wanted her father. That was why she married Gustav Mahler. The data? Alma's stepfather's name was Moll; Gustav's name was Mahler. Moll-Mahler. Does that sound less sophomoric in the original German? It must. Had her stepfather been named Bruch, would she have seduced Bruckner? That would certainly have changed his Ninth Symphony. What do you think all those drawn out repetitious climaxes in Bruckner were really about? Holy meditation? Musings on the Gospels? Or wet dreams of Alma? And those drawn out Brucknerian climaxes? It's enough to make you want to hear all eleven Bruckner symphonies. And think of having written those crescendos. Having experienced them first hand, so to speak. And Mahler himself— after all, this was his analysis. Mahler had a fixation on his mother. Who didn't? Freud had just published his famous analysis of da Vinci based on *no* hours of direct contact. He'd analyzed da Vinci's dream—a dream about a vulture. What did it matter that the Italian word that Freud translated as vulture actually didn't mean vulture at all but meant kite and that the free association was all done by Freud, not da Vinci? And Freud had also analyzed da Vinci's first anatomic drawings—the first page from Leonardo's notebooks—a hemisection of two figures during intercourse. But Freud didn't study the original drawings, he studied reproductions—reproductions that were an "improved" version of the originals—without Leonardo's notes or his other accompanying sketches.

If Freud could analyze Leonardo from such material, four hours with Mahler was bound to be sufficient, if not a downright excess of time. That done, Mahler was cured and the Mahlers lived happily ever after until he died a year later. According to Sigmund. According to Alma, nothing changed. According to history, Freud saw Mahler's obituary and sent a bill to the executors of Mahler's estate—an act that may tell us more about Freud than it does about either Gustav or Alma Mahler.

David is now after a picture of Lou Andreas Salome. And who was she? Not the inspiration for Strauss' opera of that name; that was based on Oscar Wilde's dirty play of the same name. Lou was sort of a second-class Alma. She had been Nietzsche's muse. He took one look at her and proposed. She studied with Freud and with Anna Freud. She was a leading lay analyst. And she was Rilke's mistress for several years. Back to Rilke. David will find her.

Roger

November 5

Dear Rob,

Do you remember Orville Bailey? I suppose you wouldn't. There is no particular reason why you should. He's a neuropathologist. You wouldn't have had much contact with him as an intern. I didn't, despite my interest in neurology. He's retired now. I really got to know him during my residency. I spent six months of my second year studying neuropathology with him. There were five of us working together in his lab. We did brain cutting with him three or four times a week. Orville was Chicago's premier neuropathologist and a peripatetic cutter of brains. Each week we cut all the brains in at least three different hospitals. During those six months we watched him cut hundreds of brains and we also studied the slides of all the cases he'd collected in a lifetime of neuropathology. And whenever someone sent him a set of slides for an opinion, and that happened every week for he was not just another neuropathologist, he was a nationally recognized authority, he'd give the slides to us to review individually and then he'd go over them for us.

One day a set of slides arrived, slides of a patient who had been in an auto accident and several days later had rapidly lapsed into unconsciousness. The neurosurgeon had done a brain biopsy and their neuropathologist wasn't certain what they had found. Was it a brain tumor? And, if so, was it benign or malignant? What was the relationship to the accident, if any? So they sent the slides to Orville and he gave them to us.

And we looked at them, all five of us. One at a time. And then we asked ourselves the same questions. Individually. Then as a group. We explored our ideas. Our interpretations. We debated. We isolated the key issues. We voted. And as we did, Dr. Bailey walked in. He watched. He listened. "Neuropathology," he pronounced, "is not a democratic process."

He's right. The correct diagnosis can never be voted on. A vote can be held, but the majority need not be right. Either in the path lab or at the bedside. Writing is a lot like that. Any creative process is. There's an analogy that can be explored.

Roger

November 8

Dear Rob,

Guess what Marty Bloom does for a living? No, he doesn't raise chickens. That's what ballplayers did in the '30s. That was always their fantasy. To retire from baseball and buy a chicken farm in Jersey. Did they all also long to become one of William Carlos Williams' patients?

We have Williams' stories of his patients but do we have their stories of him? Their versions? We should. Many of his patients are still alive. They must have stories about him. Has anyone ever tried to survey them? Was Williams there when they needed him? Really there? In the way he was really needed? Am I? Don't ask me.

Back to Martin Bloom, one-time major league pitcher. Any guesses, my friend? That's right. He sells insurance.

What else? I guess he could have opened a sporting goods store. Today he'd do that. Forty years ago sporting goods were not big business. Remember that was when tennis shoes were sneakers. And you wore the same sneakers for everything. Baseball, tennis, basketball. You name it. And they weren't even called cross trainers.

How did I find out? Not from his lawyer. Or mine. Or Burt's. Who may be mine. Or is mine, once removed. Someone did an article on the two of us in *The Reader*—Chicago's answer to *The Village Voice*. *The Reader*, or their reporter, at least, was intrigued by the idea of an obscure (his word, not mine) baseball player suing someone who wanted to pay tribute to his living memory. So they ran a story of the Bloom affair.

According to the story, Marty sells insurance. What else? And death is probably bad for his business. His and his clients. But publicity is supposed to be good for his business. Very good. It gives him visibility. Fame.

And they spelled his name right. And mine.

My lawyer is pissed at me. I guess I said some things to the reporter I should not have. So now I'm under orders not to talk to any reporters. Are you a reporter in disguise?

Roger

November 15

Dear Rob,

I have sent out another scientific article of sorts. In this one, I have proposed a three strike rule for scientific papers. So that each author only gets to submit each article three times. Three strikes and back to the drawing board. Or the lab. Or the word processor. No more 1.000 batting averages. No more journals stuffed with rejected articles. Here's the article:

> *To the Editor of Journal Y:*
>
> *I am often asked to contrast the scientific and literary worlds. After all, I should be an expert, having achieved some degree of success as an author in both spheres. Medically, I have published over three hundred articles and written or edited scores of books, while in my other life I have published three novels (one of which was a Book-of-the-Month Club alternate selection). The most significant difference relates to a single contrast in attitudes, a difference that, I am afraid, reflects badly on science.*
>
> *Literature is a world of rejection. Science is a world of acceptance. I am a far more "successful" writer than most, yet I have written seven novels and only three of them have ever found a home. Four remain unwanted, unaccepted by any publisher, and, hence, unpublished. While 3 out of 7 may not be a bad batting average—.429—the highest lifetime batting average of any baseball player is that of Ty Cobb—.367....*

November 20

Dear Rob,

That story about the great Walter Birkmayer has caused me a great deal of trouble. As a direct result of having written it, I've lost any number of friends. I'm sure I will lose more. Actually, it was living through the story that caused the problem more than writing it. Once having done that, I had no choice but to write and publish it. Although now that I've published it, I may have made a few more enemies. I'm glad *MD* published it. That might even be the right place. *Commentary* turned it down. So did the *New York Times*. And *Tikun*. And countless others. So I did what I always do. I converted it from a literary venture into a medical article. It is about a doctor, after all. And you know Kramer's law. All medical articles find a home. So I knew that that article was destined to find its place in the sun. So I sent it off to *MD*.

And the result? Just as I predicted. Just as my law predicted. An acceptance. If it hadn't been *MD*, there were other journals on my list. Lots of them. If you submit the same article to one journal each month, you can never run out of journals for there is at least one started each month. Think about that. That may be almost as great a threat as Birkmayer was.

Not quite.

Yes, I was shocked to discover that Birkmayer had been an SS officer during the Holocaust. I've known him for over twenty years. He's made great contributions to my field. Three contributions: perhaps the three most important ones in the last forty years. He was the first one to use levodopa. He and Andre Barbeau. Independently. At the same time. Birkmayer was also the first one to use levodopa in the form we now use it. And he was the first to say that Eldepryl may have had an effect on the course of the disease, that Eldepryl may prolong the life of patients with Parkinson's disease. That's what got the PSG started. At least in part. But he was an SS officer. A doctor in the SS. A part of the Holocaust. A cog in its machinery. Once I discovered that truth, what choice did I have? He played a role. What role? An important one, I'm sure. How can I be certain?

Had he not played his role, and had no one else played theirs, it could not have taken place. A simple truth. And truth carries a burden. And all truths are not equal. Some are more equal than others, especially in the burden they carry.

Did you see *Berlin Alexanderplatz* when it was on public television? I just discovered that the author was a neurologist. Alfred Doblin. A German Jew trained in Berlin. Eventually he went into practice there. He finally gave up medicine to become a writer. And fled Germany, of course. First to France and then to the United States. Here he converted to Catholicism and tried to make a living writing for the movies.

Another marginal tragic figure. More outsider than insider. His last book has just been translated into English. It's called *Destiny's Journey*. It is about his experiences fleeing himself and the Nazis and then, after the war, returning to Germany as an officer with the French occupying forces. He was in charge of de-Nazifying German literature. A time for looking into his own soul once again.

Günter Grass was his disciple.

Perhaps I should send a copy to Birkmayer. Perhaps in German. Perhaps not.

Roger

November 21

Dear Rob,

Your story reaches its climax because of a coincidence. You can't do that.

Climaxes don't come about like that. You should know that. Nature abhors coincidence. No, it's not nature that abhors any coincidence. It's editors who abhor coincidences. Editors and scientists. Nature thrives on coincidence. Nature doesn't even recognize it as coincidence. Coincidence is random activity at work. It is the expression of chaos. Of unpredictability. Of uncertainty. Hence, it is not coincidental. It is not the remarkable co-occurrence of events. It is their co-occurrence but there is nothing at all remarkable about that. Nothing out of the ordinary. Nothing coincidental about coincidence.

That's what science is all about. The whole damn scientific method. And all the statistics we use. The management of randomness. All those damn biostatisticians we employ. The ones who determined that we needed eight hundred patients to study Eldepryl and who knew the exact moment when we'd reached statistical significance. That it wasn't coincidence. That Eldepryl was active. It was doing something other than increasing the value of Mylan's stock. That's science.

Science may start off with a coincidence. A happenstance. An observation. With a capital O. But is that observation an observation? Was what was observed merely a random event? A coincidence? Or part of the organized function of the world, an expression of scientific fact?

Science at work. From event to truth. Let's make a hypothesis. We'll call it a null hypothesis. Why null? Because its purpose is to be proven null and void. And null sounds better than void.

So what's our hypothesis? That the observation, the apparent fact that A and B occurred together, took place because they do occur together by design, not by random chance. Not by the happenstance of chaos. Nothing random here. The hypothesis is set. I know we test it the other way around, by assuming, by hypothesizing randomness and then seeing how likely or unlikely that is. Next comes the experiment. Isolating A and B in some other setting.

Collecting the data.

Analyzing it.

Running a statistical test. What does that tell you? Whether the observed coincidence of A and B was due to random variance. Coincidence. Chaos. Or by design. That's all statistics tell us. And the design of the experiment is what counts. Only if the design is valid do the statistics mean anything at all. Beauty is in the design. Beauty and truth.

A good experiment controls all the variables. It can be run over and over again. And you can then analyze whether your result was just an observation of chaos. Mere chance. At a five percent level. One out of twenty. Or, better, a one percent level. One out of a hundred. Ninety-nine out of one hundred. It wasn't chance. Null has not been nulled. Experimental science is one long exercise in controlling coincidence. And to run statistics, to test the variables, you have to be able to measure those variables. To count them. And if they are clinical variables, you must have a scale. A scale that works. That other scientists use and understand and trust. The trust is in the scale.

Why didn't Garcia use a real scale? A known scale? A proven scale? He used his own scale? Is it trustworthy? Is it valid? Is it reliable? Is he? Does his scale control coincidence? Does he?

He must. He's trying to be a scientist and that is what scientists do all day long.

And so must writers. One coincidence is okay if done correctly. If it's the original observation. A coincidence that launches a thousand ships is okay. It passes muster. Hitchcock understood that. More than anyone. He starts off each movie with a coincidence. An observation. His hero is in the wrong place at the wrong time and sees something. What? Even the hero isn't sure. It was a coincidence. But after that there are no more coincidences. Nothing else is random, no matter how chaotic it seems. That Piper Cub flying overhead to spray the corn field is no coincidence. Cary Grant knew that. So did each and every moviegoer. One coincidence per film. One coincidence per customer. And that's if you're writing a thriller. Which no true writer should be doing. There are no coincidences in *The Third Man*. It is the coincidence that three friends of Harry Limes are all there at his "death" that proves it was not a coincidence. That's what makes it a great story. I almost wrote great "literature."

But if a coincidence does happen in literature, it must serve a purpose. What purpose? Irony. That's what differentiates literature from thrillers. The conversion of coincidence into irony makes it literature.

Coincidences do happen in life. They happen in science. If you run one hundred experiments at the one percent level, one of them will be significant at the one percent level as a result of mere chance.

But which one? That's the rub.

And five at the five percent level. Which is too damn many rubs to deal with.

Coincidence occurs. Seeing your best friend's wife go into a motel with a man who is not your best friend is just that. A coincidence. Not an act of God. Not an act that gives meaning to life. What you do with that observation may be, but not the observation itself. What you do with the incidental observation is what counts. It is what makes someone a scientist and someone else a writer and the rest of us merely bystanders. Or troublemakers.

Roger

November 24

Dear Rob,

The burden of David's Holocaust story was not easily surmounted. Telling it was a most difficult task. Perhaps the most difficult of my entire literary career. Perhaps of my entire career. I had no idea at all as to what I should do. How I should get started. In science that's always been easy. The problem is obvious. So is the goal. The secret is in the method. Ask the right question. A simple one. One that can be tested. Nothing Freudian. Nothing untestable. What to do? David had given me the story and the charge to tell that story. It was much more than a charge. It was almost a sacred obligation. I had to tell the story. It was like writing about Birkmayer. I had no choice in either matter. But how to do it?

I had just finished a novel then. My fourth. It was my first without my alter hero, Paul Richardson. It was an international spy/thriller set in Paris, Chicago, Amsterdam, Syria, Jerusalem. The hero was a disaffected Dutchman who was intentionally cast as an outsider. Not your classic innocent hero who by coincidence gets involved in some devious plot or other. Not Cary Grant in the wrong place. Nor James Stewart and Doris Day. Or Grace Kelly. Or Kim Novak. Nothing out of Hitchcock. Nor Helen MacInnes. Not even Eric Ambler.

My hero would be no one's choice for a hero. Even mine. Except he was. He is. In the first third of the book he is all but downright despicable, in the middle third he becomes sympathetic, and then in the last third truly heroic. In a classic sense. The rest of the details are superfluous. The how's and why's of these transitions cannot be summarized in a scant paragraph or two. If they could, what would have justified an entire novel? The book was done. More than done. It had already been rejected by half a dozen publishers.

So I revised it. I didn't change my protagonist. I did buff him up a bit, but not too much. And I added David's story as part of the Amsterdam background. So much for my obligation. I had performed it. I'd done what David had asked me to do.

Twenty rejection slips later, I knew I had not discharged my duty. Putting that story into an unsold manuscript was not enough. Especially if it remained unsold.

Back to the beginning.

What to do?

I was into being a playwright then. Did I ever really think I would be a playwright? Probably not. But think of the milieu. Each Saturday, another reading. A room filled with would-be playwrights. All of whom were trying to make progress on a work in progress. Seeing a work in progress. Dissecting it. Analyzing it. And then once every four months or so, it's my Saturday afternoon.

Mine. My own work in progress. A director, actors, actresses. Rehearsals. Discussions. Changes. Input. Serious input. Input as dialogue. Not by someone with one eye on sales and the other on marketing. Creative criticism. And then the reading in front of a live audience.

Almost orgasmic.

I happened to read a play by Ayckbourn. One of his less successful ones. *Couples*. Don't feel bad, most people have never heard of it. One of the scenes takes place in a restaurant. And all you can hear is what the waiter hears. What a brilliant concept. A great piece of stagecraft.

I stole it. That idea. That concept. I almost called it *What the Waiter Heard*. After that the entire play wrote itself.

Table one: The doctor. The one who does examinations on survivors under contract from the German government. And with him the doctor's wife. With a lot of tension between the two of them. Two different people with the doctor as philanderer. Like so many doctors we both know.

Table two: The survivor, who has just been examined by the doctor who was under contract from the German government, and his overprotective daughter.

One coincidence. Same restaurant. Not so bad. It's down the block from the doctor's office. Not that much of a coincidence.

The tables are at opposite sides of the stage. The waiter goes from table to table. We hear what he hears. No more, no less. He, of course, never reacts. He hears without hearing. Sees without observing. History does not involve him. It happens around him. He is a waiter. That is not his day job, that is what he is.

Once the conceit is set, the personalities tell the story. The doctor. The survivor. Two versions of history. Coming together with a single line. That line is said as the waiter for the first time goes directly from table two to table one. The only direct bridge in the play.

Father: The mumzer. He said that they. . . .

Doctor: . . . don't pay for dreams. Ha! Ha!

The father leaves. So does the wife. And the daughter tries to pick up the doctor, who realizes who she is and turns her down.

CURTAIN.

I was done. I'd fulfilled my obligation. Not the first time. That was a disaster. The old man was played by a nice, retired, gentile school teacher who butchered the accent and never got the word "mumzer" out at all. But the second time it worked.

One hundred percent. Even David said so. The title was *Dinner for Two at David's*. Or *Dinner for Two* for short.

The second time was part of a festival of plays in progress. We staged it twice. Two separate readings. I'd done it. I'd gotten the message out. To fewer than one hundred people. Not exactly mass communication.

That was my last staged reading. By then *Toscanini* had been sold in the U.K., the Netherlands, Germany, Japan, Spain. And I had a big contract for the next book. So I gave up show biz. Milieu is not all. Perhaps a tree in a forest, an empty forest, makes a noise. But who the hell cares?

Roger

One-act play with five characters: Two older men in their sixties. One older woman in her fifties. One woman in her late twenties. One man of any age. Or no specific age. Length: Thirty minutes. Full script available from the author.

November 27

Dear Rob,

Don't underestimate Alan Ayckbourn, and certainly don't undervalue his contribution to theater. Although, being an American, it would be rather difficult not to. You could start by not judging him by those terrible puns he uses as titles. *Absurd Person Singular* or *Relatively Speaking*. You can not judge a playwright by the words that appear on the marquee. In my view he is the best playwright around these days because he understands theater and its conventions and traditions and prejudices and conceits and can turn these all around and use them so that the artifice becomes the reality.

And why is he such a good playwright?

Probably because he quit school at seventeen and started working in the theater. Backstage. Shakespeare, I remind you, was not college-educated.

Ayckbourn has now written more plays than Shakespeare, even if you count all those dreadful early ones. By Shakespeare, not Ayckbourn. His early works certainly stand up better than the Bard's, but then he had the advantage of having worked on his, Shakespeare's, later plays before he wrote his own earlier ones. Shakespeare never had that opportunity.

My favorite is his trilogy, *The Norman Conquests*. Another pun. It's not about William the Conqueror. It's about Norman the would-be conqueror. The conquistador of women. It consists of three plays with no specific set order. No chronology. No historical record to be preserved. They all involve the same six characters: Norman. His wife. His brother-in-law. His brother-in-law's wife. His brother and his sister-in-law. Nice and symmetrical, that. They, the three plays, all take place during the same time frame, a single weekend.

What unity. Aristotle would have loved it.

Unity of person.

Unity of time.

Unity of place.

With subunits. Here is where Ayckbourn's particular genius comes into play. The first play, *Table Manners*, is all of the action, all of the conversations, all of the interactions that take place around the dining room table—in other words, whatever could be seen, heard, felt, or otherwise observed in the dining room during that three-day weekend.

A producer's dream—a single set. And a single story. With a beginning, a middle, and an end. A complete play that stands by itself. The story of an attempted conquest by Norman. His brother-in-law's wife. Or his sister-in-law. I forget which. That doesn't matter.

Play two: Same characters. Same weekend. Same house. Same unities. Different artifice. Different room. Different title. *Living Together*. The living room. Or, as the stage directions say, the sitting room. Everything that happened that weekend in a different room. The story of a separate room, a separate seduction. The second of Norman's conquests. And a complete play whole unto itself. With all those unities. And again a single set.

Play three: You guessed it. Same people. Same weekend. Same house. Same chase. Different object. His wife, I think. Different set. The garden. *Round and Round the Garden*. Each is a complete play. You can see one or two or three and in any order, but three, all three, the sum of experiencing all three is greater than the sum of its three parts. One plus one plus one is more than three. The new math.

If I ever write a trilogy, an idea with which I have toyed, that would be my model. Not *The Forsythe Saga*. Not some cave dwellers. Not a family traced generation to generation. But one person. One character. My own Norman. Not *Rashamon*. Not looking at the same action from three different perspectives. But three sets of actions in one man's life. His profession. His passionate avocation. His private life. Not intertwined but segregated so that each can be fully and separately dissected. Each a complete story. And, believe me, one plus one plus one would certainly be more than three.

There is one big problem. Is a trilogy one at bat or three? If I submit a trilogy, does that count as one attempt or three? A dilemma.

I'm sure Alan Ayckbourn would know how to solve it. And perhaps one of our biostatisticians.

I got a letter from one of the physiatrists today, a geriatric physiatrist no less. She takes care of a lot of our parkinson patients in the geriatric rehabilitation facility. Her letter was about one of my parkinson patients who had just completed six weeks of in-patient rehabilitation. The patient, the letter said, was much improved. He had made great progress. Many, many gains. Shades of Sam Levinson.

You remember Sam Levinson. Or maybe you don't. He was a stand-up comedian in the early days of TV. The '50s. His original day job had been as a high school teacher/principal. In that job he'd written untold numbers of letters of recommendation for students applying for college. Then he got a letter back from the Dean of Admissions at NYU: "Dear Mr. Levinson," the letter began. "You have now recommended four hundred leaders of the future to us. Please send one follower." Has not at least one of my patients made only modest gains? Or none at all? Don't ask. We both know the answer.

It all reminds me of my favorite consult request. It asked simply, "Can you help this patient?" I saw the patient. I took a history. I did an examination. I reviewed the chart. I wrote my consult.

"No!" No euphemism. No beating around the bush. No equivocations.

Roger

P. S. Ayckbourn described his Chekhov period as the time when nothing happened in his plays, very slowly. How could he not be a genius?

December

The major difference between good doctors and bad doctors is that good doctors remember every mistake they ever made. We all make mistakes sooner or later, sometimes serious ones. You can't make the kind of decisions we make day after day, night after night, sometimes all night long, without being wrong sometimes. The good doctors remember, the others don't. Maybe they don't care, maybe they need to forget, maybe they did it too often. But they don't remember.

Harold L. Klawans
Sins of Commission

Monday, December 2

Dear Rob:

I'm sorry I haven't gotten around to writing you for four or five days, but I've been extremely busy. Do you realize that that was my first ordinary excuse since I got started on this routine? Ordinary events, like ordinary characters, have so little literary merit. Which makes literature like medicine. The study of the abnormal, the grotesque. Not of the normal. The normal may well be the stuff that science is made of, but not medicine or literature. We live in a world of disease, not of health.

This weekend we hosted a national meeting of most of the investigators who are performing adrenal implants on Parkinson's disease patients. We invited everybody: neurologists, neurosurgeons, laboratory scientists, the kind of people who haven't been out of their labs in twenty years. The meeting was held here in Chicago.

My associate, Arnold Chiari, and I did most of the organizing. Arnold has pretty much taken over the administration of our research program, both literally and officially. And none too soon. That leaves me more time to write letters to you, and maybe even a novel or two. What have you given up lately?

Arnold presented the results on our first four patients. They are all improved. Not cured, mind you. Not a trip to Lourdes amongst them. Not a quadrat of miracles, but their Parkinson's disease is less bothersome, less disabling. They all have more "on" time and less "off" time. More good time; less bad time, and the bad time is not as bad as it used to be, for any one of them. Take patient four for instance. She's pretty typical of what we've observed. Instead of a pair of two hour periods each day during which she was immobile, her "off" phases now last only an hour apiece and during them she can still walk by herself. And she no longer has to end her day at six. She can stay up until nine or ten. She hasn't done that in years. Her "on" time is not much better than it was, but even before surgery that had been pretty good.

But what does it all mean, Rob? That's the key issue. It's only been a couple of months. And we only have seen these results in a few patients. A few patients do not a revolution make.

A number of other groups also presented their early results. Some were similar to ours. Others were a litany of surgical disasters, of operative mortalities, of post-operative complications. Of deaths. Of permanent neurologic catastrophes. Most of those problems occurred at places with no previous experience in treating patients with Parkinson's disease. Places that only became interested in Parkinson's disease because of Garcia and all the hoopla. What right did they have to operate on these patients in the first place? I'm not questioning their legal right. I'm questioning their ethical right. They don't know how to take care of such patients. All right, I'll get off my high horse.

All in all, the meeting was a success. Most surgeons are beginning to realize they need us poor neurologists to take care of the patients and to tell them if the implant really worked. And the world does, too. How is that for grandiosity?

Roger

December 3

Dear Randy,

Congratulations on a job well done. It was not only the right thing to do, but it will also save me money. A legal rarity, that—saving the client money. I'm relieved that Tinker agreed to allow you to carry the ball, to let you and your office do all the legal work in regard to *Bloom vs. Kramer et al*. What a relief. No reduplication of effort. No double billing of me. But is that how the law is supposed to work?

Roger

December 4

Dear Rob,

You are not the only one who reads *MD*. Thank God. I wanted that story to reach people. I wanted people to read it. I still do. I hope at least some of the subscribers leave copies in their reception rooms. Their waiting rooms. Where patients sit and wait. And sometimes read. Right there with *People* magazine and *National Geographic*.

Some people have read it and have even taken the time to write letters to me. One was a man, a survivor, who had gone to gymnasium with Knoll, the man who discovered Eldepryl. They grew up in Budapest. That was in the '30s, before the war. They were both Hungarian Jews. And they were both saved by Raoul Wallenberg. The writer of the letter came to the United States in '56, when Russia sent in the tanks to crush the freedom movement in Hungary. He's a physician. He's retired now. According to his friend, Knoll was more a pharmacologist than a physician. He stayed in Hungary. He is still living there, alive and well. Knoll invented Eldepryl not to treat Parkinson's disease, but as an antidepressant. It was Birkmayer who first used it in PD. With Knoll's blessings, I'm sure.

Did Knoll know about Birkmayer? That was what his old classmate wondered in his letter to me. Does he know now? If not, he will very soon. The classmate was about to send him a copy of my article. So soon Knoll will read it.

Will Birkmayer? Will someone send him a copy? Will Birkmayer then sue me? And, if so, for what? For libel? Of course, he'll have to get in line behind Marty Bloom. Could they somehow make it into a class action suit? Will Birkmayer actually pull an Oscar Wilde and take me to court? Wilde, you will recall, was a free man writing away and being himself until he sued the Marquis of Queensbury for libel. The libel? Calling Wilde a sodomist. Truth is a defense. Wilde lost. And the police then had no choice but to arrest Wilde. Sodomy was illegal in England. An illegal act that called for stern punishment. So Wilde sued and ended up in jail. Or, as he put it, in "gaol." Yes, he got a book out of the experience. That's what writers do. All things considered, it wasn't worth it. Better he should have written a far different book.

Another letter was far more troublesome. It was also from a physician whose name I will withhold for the sake of his family. It was not even a letter. It was a postcard.

"There were good Jews and bad Jews," he began. "Were there not good SS officers?"

Good Jews! Bad Jews! What did bad mean? Nonobservant? Eating ham sandwiches on Passover? Or good in the minds of their oppressors?

Good SS officers! What a concept. What a notion. What did it mean? That they followed orders well. Genug!

You say that you want to write a novel. Isn't this a good enough plot for you? Not my story. Write me out of it. I can be like da Ponte in *Amadeus*. Knoll's story. The story of a survivor whose one discovery becomes significant because of the efforts of an ex-SS officer. Eldepryl was never a great antidepressant. It was never even marketed in this country. Now it is a neurological revolution. All because of the work of one unrepentant Nazi. Any ordinary experience? God forbid.

Pathos enough? Irony enough? Or just reality?

Another of those daily coincidences.

Today is an anniversary of sorts. On this date in 1580 the Inquisition condemned Garcia d'Orta to be burned as a heretic. Garcia d'Orta was the greatest of all Portuguese physicians until this century. A great name in the history of medicine. He lived and worked in Genoa. He wrote the first pharmacopoeia, the first textbook on medications since the second century. A landmark achievement. But, alas, he was a secret Jew. His forced conversion had not taken. He had lapsed back into Judaism. He was a heretic. And so he was condemned to be burned. An *auto da fé*.

The only problem was that by the time the Inquisition pronounced its holy sentence, d'Orta had been dead for a dozen years. No matter. Dig up the bones and burn them. Which is precisely what was done.

Such a man should be honored. And such craziness should be remembered.

Roger

December 4

Dear Doctor Whose Name Is Being Withheld Out of Respect for His Family,
    Name three.

> Roger Kramer
> *Professor of Neurology*

cc: Rob

December 6

Dear Rob,
    I was flicking channels last night. That's what's so great about cable TV; there are so many more channels to choose not to watch. That's real democracy in action. Voting with your remote control. And each choice was so easy to make. As easy as voting against Richard Nixon. Or for whoever was running against him. McGovern. So there I was clicking away until I got to WGN and *IT* was on. The Great American Movie. The Great American Screenplay. It was quickly coming to a climax. Ingrid Bergman and her husband, Victor Laslow, papers in hand, were already on the plane to fly off to Portugal and from there to the West to continue their fight against Hitler. Who could be opposed to that? Then or now? The plane was slowly beginning to taxi through the early evening fog of the Casablanca airport. Rick, a.k.a. Humphrey Bogart, stands there in his trench coat, his right hand in his pocket holding a pistol pointed at Captain Renault, the Prefect of Police, to make sure that nothing goes wrong.
    But it does. Colonel Strasser, head of the SS in Casablanca, arrives, having been surreptitiously called by Renault. Renault, who somehow comes out of this as, well, if not a hero, at least a pretty good guy, tells Strasser what is happening. The plane is beginning its takeoff, to take Laslow to freedom, to continue his fight. Our fight. The world's fight.
    Strasser grabs the phone to call the tower.
    Rick tells him to put the phone down.
    Strasser refuses. He must stop Laslow. It's his job. And he is good at his job. Good, not bad.

He was willing to shoot Renault, Rick warns Strasser. He is certainly willing to kill Strasser, the SS officer. The epitome of evil. A good SS officer, through and through.

Strasser, a Nazi to the end, pulls out his gun, so Rick shoots him. Strasser is dead. His body slumps to the floor. The plane continues its takeoff, but is still on the ground. A car filled with French gendarmes arrives, called previously by the now late Colonel Strasser.

This is it. The moment of truth. Recall the scene. Strasser is on the floor, dead. Rick is standing there, smoking gun in hand. And the only witness is the Prefect of Police himself, Captain Renault. Claude Raines. Never a man to be trusted. He'd proved his untrustfulness in a score of previous film roles. The police size up the situation and turn to their Captain for orders. Renault, good ol' Claude Raines, comes through.

"Colonel Strasser has been shot," he announces, and then, resurrecting a line from the opening sequence of the movie following the murder of the German courier for the famous letters of transit, Renault tells his men to "round up the usual suspects." Good writing, that. Bringing back a familiar line. Bringing it all together so neatly.

And what a line! *The usual suspects.*

Ignore the smoking gun. Round up the usual suspects. Rick and Renault watch the plane complete its takeoff and then walk off in the mist to join a Free French garrison and begin a beautiful friendship. That Free French garrison, by the way, is in the Belgian Congo, a mere several hundred miles away. A fairly long walk, that.

Perhaps Renault is truly a hero. And the movie is a work of art. And that line of Colonel Renault's all too memorable. But to me it is all too descriptive of the way most scientists whom I know and whose work floods the journals I used to read so conscientiously spend their lives: *lining up the usual suspects.*

Then today in the office, I was again reminded of the same phenomenon. A patient of mine, a fairly new patient at that, had asked me to recommend a hypnotist to him to help control his Parkinson's disease. He's a young man, about forty-five, with mild Parkinson's.

I refused.

"Why?" he asked me.

I told him that I never recommend anything to a patient that does not have a proven value. If hypnotism is to be used to treat Parkinson's disease patients, it was the job of those who bill such patients to prove that their product, their service, works. Drug companies have to do that.

Now even surgeons do. Why not hypnotists? Why not acupuncturists for that matter?

It was not the answer he had expected to get. He changed the subject. He wanted to know how research worked. How did scientists learn about Parkinson's disease? All to be explained while standing on one foot. "By lining up the usual suspects," I said. He had no idea what I meant. I started again. "Look, most scientists aren't Einsteins. They make progress by applying new techniques to old problems and that is not much more than just the routine of application of the scientific approach."

He still had no idea what I was talking about.

I tried to explain by giving him an example. I talked about dopamine. It was the one brain chemical that he already knew something about. I started by telling him that dopamine had been known to exist in the brain for many years, but until the mid '50s there was no good way to measure it. Then someone developed a method, so it got measured in the brains of rats. And it was discovered to be only in certain areas of the brain, not equally distributed everywhere. But was that true in humans, too? Another scientist used that same technique and found the same uneven distribution of dopamine.

So what? Did that mean anything? No one knew, but one area with a very high concentration was a part of the brain that some people thought might play a role in diseases like Parkinson's disease. So someone else, using this same technique, started measuring dopamine in the brains of patients who had died with various neurologic diseases. That was what Oleh Hornekiewicz did. In Vienna in the late '50s and early '60s. He worked with Birkmayer. Did he know? If so, when? And did he forget? Dopamine was normal in Huntington's disease, in epilepsy, in multiple sclerosis, but not in Parkinson's disease. It was low in Parkinson's disease. Very low. Hornekiewicz had lined up the suspects and located the one with the smoking gun.

My patient seemed to understand. "But that is not how you do research," he smiled at me.

It was time for another story. I told him the saga of the bouncing guinea pigs, my infamous popcorn pigs. While in Europe one summer, 1971, I think, it occurred to me that I did not know what happened to behavior when we increased another chemical in the brain called serotonin. That is not such a peculiar notion, or a very insightful one either. Too little dopamine causes parkinsonism. Too much causes abnormal behaviors. My lab did a lot of research on those behaviors related to increasing the brain dopamine levels. If we increased the related chemical, serotonin, was some sort of abnormal behavior produced? So later that night I called Chicago to talk to one of the medical students who was working in my laboratory. This student had been interested in finding a simple project that she could do on her own, and when I had left for Vienna, I hadn't yet come up with one, but promised her I would continue to think about it. Well, now I had the idea. I told her to give 5-HTP to guinea pigs to see what would happen. 5-HTP is the precursor of serotonin. If you give it to an animal, the brain level of serotonin will increase.

"What *will* happen?" she asked.

"I have no idea," I replied.

"Then why should we do it?"

"To see what will happen. That's called research."

"Why guinea pigs? Why not rats? Rats are less expensive."

"Two reasons," I explained. We knew more about the chemistry of the guinea pig and much more about their normal behaviors. "Besides, I hate rats," I added. Like the hero of *1984,* whatever his name was. Good ol' Orwell. That is another part of *1984* that I remember. Those rats. How I hated them. How he hated them. And was afraid of them. And they knew it. Big Brother knew it. What was his name? Who knows? Who remembers? That is why I would not have chosen Orwell.

It took about twenty minutes more for me to outline the various experiments that had to be set up, and by the time I was done, she, too, was interested in the project.

I didn't get back to Chicago and my laboratory for over a month. When I did, the woman whom I had talked to from Vienna collared me immediately. "The guinea pigs," she said, "they bounce like kernels of popcorn."

This I had to see.

I watched as she injected some normal guinea pigs with 5-HTP. For the first five minutes, nothing happened. The earliest abnormal behavior that I saw was some increased grooming behavior. The animals appeared to brush their faces and scratch their sides with their paws, at first off and on and then continuously. Just when the grooming behavior peaked, the second behavioral alteration began: a sudden shaking or jerking of the head and neck. These jerks also began sporadically, but they quickly became continuous and almost rhythmic. Then the most impressive behavior started. They did bounce. It was a peculiar rhythmic bouncing of the whole animal. The animals appeared to jump straight up from the floor of the cage, often propelled forward or backward. Often the guinea pigs had all four feet off the floor at the same time.

I was impressed. Did all the animals bounce?

That depended on the dose of 5-HTP they had been given. At 100 mg., none bounced; at 200 mg., one out of four bounced; and at 300 mg., they all bounced. The frequency of the bouncing was also dose-related: at 300 mg., the guinea pigs bounced at a rate of sixty bounces per minute; at 400 mg., they bounced at a rate of eighty to one hundred bounces per minute.

"What should we do next?" the student asked.

"We'll measure the effect of 5-HTP on brain serotonin levels and see if the bouncing correlates with the elevation in brain serotonin."

"Anything else?"

"Don't give it to any elephants."

Two weeks later, at our weekly laboratory meeting, the student presented the results. 5-HTP did increase brain serotonin, just as I had expected. More important, the degree of that increase in serotonin was related to the severity of the bouncing behavior.

So now we had a way of observing and quantifying one effect of serotonin in the brain of a healthy animal and we knew one thing that serotonin did: it caused bouncing, whatever that meant.

An animal model of popcorn, she suggested.

Her reply was not as sarcastic as it sounds. My laboratory spent most of its efforts in those years studying animal behaviors as models of human diseases. Here we had a behavior without a disease, a model without a home. Like a cure without an illness. It was not much good to anyone. I was the clinician, the specialist in human behaviors, normal and abnormal. It was my job to find the human analogy.

About one week later, I walked into the laboratory just as the injected guinea pigs were at the height of their grooming behavior, before they had commenced the head jerks or bouncing. I dropped a heavy medical book on the table next to the observation cage, and it slapped down with a sharp thud. The pigs bounced, all six of them, one single bounce each, and all six at the same time.

I lifted up the book again and dropped it. Thud. All six guinea pigs bounced up off the floor of the cage.

Each time I dropped the book, a sudden bounce of six experimental animals followed.

"Stimulus-sensitive bouncing," I said.

"So?" came the response from my student.

"It's the perfect animal model of the jumping Frenchmen of Maine."

"Of what?" she asked.

I tried to explain. The "jumping Frenchmen of Maine" was the name given to a neurologic disorder that had been described in some French trappers who lived in Maine in the 1880s. Sudden noises caused them to jump.

Had I ever seen such a patient? No.

Had anyone I ever knew seen one? No.

She thought I should keep looking for my human analogy. A model of a disease no one had seen since the nineteenth century was unlikely to change the course of American neurology.

So I did just that. I rounded up the usual suspects. One at a time. All of the movement disorders characterized by sudden stimulus-sensitive jerks. I started with the more common ones and worked my way down the usual list, striking out with a regularity that became so monotonous that our efforts ground to a halt.

Why? Time is not infinite. Nor money. And research takes both. I was 0 for 21. It was time to go on. None of the usual subjects were guilty. So what? No big deal. Just another in a long list of unsolved mysteries. After all, the murder of Colonel Strasser is still unsolved.

It was only two years later that I found the smoking gun in the guise of a young girl, not yet two years old, who jerked and jumped like a kernel of popcorn because of a tumor in her abdomen, called a neuroblastoma, a tumor made up of nerve cells that could and did make lots of neurochemicals, including 5-HTP.

I had found the smoking gun. Rick had been holding it all the time. I'd just been busy rounding up the usual suspects. Science at work.

Roger

December 10

Dear Rob,
STRIKE TWO!
"Ain't my style," said Casey.

Turned down again. Another called strike. My bat was still on my shoulder. I never even got a decent swing. Two submissions, two rejections. This one even came with a letter, an editorial letter, telling my agent that I'm a good writer and that *The Blind Observer* is a good book. But a novel on AIDS just wouldn't fit on their list. FIT ON THEIR LIST! What the hell does that mean? Other than strike two?

At least I'll be out of the batter's box for a while. What with Christmas coming on, my agent is not going to submit it to any other publishers until January. Then he'll send it to three at the same time.

Which three? His choice, not mine. He's sharpening his darts. Let's hope he throws a strike. Now that's a mixed metaphor. Throws a bull's-eye. Either will do.

Of course, I had another paper accepted today. This is the one the *New England Journal* turned down. And *Neurology*. So it's in *Archives*. It's still a publication. My four hundred and eleventh. Four hundred and eleven out of four hundred and eleven. Maintaining my 1.000 batting average. Just like everyone else. That makes me average. Just plain mediocre. In fact, in this field, I cannot get above mediocre. Nor can you. Or anyone else. Ain't that a pisser?

I'd assumed you knew that Orwell had died of tuberculosis, although I'm not sure why I made that assumption. It seems as if I've always known it. Long before I knew precisely what tuberculosis was and far before I knew that it was, in most otherwise healthy people, a treatable disease. A curable disease.

You are right to be surprised. It's not surprising to learn that Chekhov died of tuberculosis. That was in turn-of-the-century Russia. And Kafka, Middle Europe in the '20's. Long before PAS and INH and streptomycin. But Orwell. He's a contemporary. He outlived the Second World War. He didn't live in Russia or Prague, but in London. Not the turn-of-the-century London of Sherlock Holmes and endless smog, but our own mid-century. Yet it was not quite as recent as all that. At least not medically. It makes you realize how quickly things can change. Five years later he might well have been cured.

When my mother was in nurses' training, her best friend went into a diabetic coma and died. And a month later the first insulin arrived in Chicago. I must have heard my mother tell that story a dozen times or more. And it took years to put it into perspective. Miracles might be just around the corner, but you can't count on that. And that never justifies prolonging suffering.

My agent and I also talked about my next project. Not this one. God forbid. This is just between the two of us at the moment. An epistilatory novel in this marketplace? I never mentioned it. And I certainly didn't bring up the notion of a trilogy. We talked about *The Return of Toscanini's Miscue*. And for the first time in my career, I now know that I am a real writer, not a scientist playing at literature, but a real writer, a true modern American author. In the tradition of. . . . Stephen Sondheim did a musical called *Merrily We Roll Along*, not one of his most successful, although it is one of my favorites. It was based on a Kaufman and Hart play of a far different name, *Once in a Life Time*. Sondheim changed the characters, the time, the setting, the story line, and added his songs, doing both the music and the lyrics. His version ends up being about a songwriting team. One of them, the lyricist, is interviewed on TV and asked which came first, the music or the lyrics? The classic question. There is no one right answer. For Rodgers and Hart, not the same Hart, Lorenz, not Moss, the music came first. Rodgers wrote the right melody for the right place in the right scene and then Hart's job was to create the right words. For Rodgers and Hammerstein, same Rodgers, the lyrics came first. Hammerstein wrote the book, the libretto, and all the lyrics and then it was Rodgers' job to make the melody fit the rhyme. Gershwin's words. Ira, not George. In opera, it has always been the words, the libretto, that came first, even with da Ponte and Mozart.

Which came first, the lyricist was asked?

"Generally," the lyricist replied, "the contract."

The modern creative artist in three words—"Generally, the contract."

And unless I get an offer, I'm not sure I'll even write *The Son of Toscanini's Miscue*. So much for artistic creativity. Maybe I'll just write my letters to you. Or my trilogy. Or both.

After all, who does unfunded research? That would be tantamount to heresy. And they even dig up the bones of heretics to burn them.

Roger

December 16

Dear Rob,

Of course, Freud bashing is easy. That is why so many people seem to do it so very well. And, of course, it's in. How could it not be both? And this situation is far more his fault than ours. He so totally immersed himself in literature and science that he lost track of where the former ended and the latter began and vice versa. That may have fit in quite well with psychoanalytic theory and dream interpretation and all that, the leaking over of dreams into wakefulness, of the unconscious into consciousness, all so nice and tidy, as long as you suppress the realities of what science is. It is an error to which I may be somewhat hypersensitive. After all, I do not want to make that same mistake. Or even be accused of it. Being sued for libel is okay. I can take that in stride. Even malpractice. But confusing my two professions, never. One must never call his wife by his mistress's name. Or the other way around either.

But Freud did. He lost track of which was which. Who was who. The rules of the game. And when you come right down to it, you can't do that. Even if you are Sigmund Freud. Karl Popper was right. The only purpose of hypothesis in science is to be proven wrong. To be able to be proven wrong, a hypothesis must be tested. To be tested, it must be testable. What in Freud is testable? The Oedipus complex? Penis envy? The interpretation of dreams? The meaning of symbols?

And it wasn't just the dream material that blurred the borders—not just his willingness to interpret faulty data to draw conclusions from secondhand inaccuracies as to what da Vinci had dreamed or even drawn. Those errors are bad enough. In a class with Garcia forgetting how many patients he had operated on. And that a couple had died. And that no one was sure what he was measuring. Am I pressing my point too far? Perhaps. The problem in relationship to Freud started right in the beginning, before the beginning—with Anna O. You remember her. She was the first case study in the *Five Case Studies of Hysteria* by Breuer and Freud. The first one. The first labor contraction in the birth of psychoanalysis. Freud's first psychoanalytic patient. His first cure.

But she had not even been Freud's patient. Not even for a wham bam four hour analysis à la Gustav Mahler. She'd been Breuer's patient a decade before. A patient treated by Breuer. Treated by him with hypnosis. Treated and cured. And cured of such symptoms. One hundred and twenty-three episodes of paralysis that could only be cured by reliving them in exact reverse chronologic order. Over a hundred periods of deafness. Again, these could only be cured by their recreation in exact reverse chronologic order. Under hypnosis, of course. Not analysis. Mesmer, not Freud.

Exact reverse chronologic order!

Order chronologic reversed exactly! Not quite a palindrome, but getting close. Who was kidding whom? No one could ever have taken that process seriously. Or believed that all that ever happened. No similar case had ever been reported before. Or since. So who was lying to whom?

Anna O. wasn't her name. Her name was Bertha Pappenheim. She became one of the founders of professional social work in Germany. A brilliant, accomplished lady. So perhaps Anna O. had lied to Breuer. Patients have lied to their doctors before Anna O. And since. Did she lie to Breuer? That's one possibility.

But that's not the only possibility here. There are more candidates. Or should I say suspects. Like Ibsen revisited. Hedda revisited. Once you believe it was murder, all sorts of suspects appear. So once you accept the inherent falsity of the story, there are lots of suspects. *Breuer!* Did he lie to Freud?

Who was Breuer? He was also a great scientist. He discovered how the inner ear works. He was a great clinician. In Vienna, he was the doctor's doctor. Was there a survey? Did they ask the same question? And get answers for the same reasons? Was he the one who lied? To Freud.

Or *Freud?* Could he have lied to us? Sigmund as liar. Not just lying to himself. But to the world.

One thing is certain. It wasn't just Anna O. How can we be sure of that? Her treatment with Breuer ended with her admission to a sanitorium. Freud and Breuer wrote that she'd been cured. Most of us do not consider institutionalization as a form of a cure. In Anna O. they also wrote about a false pregnancy. But what really had happened? Breuer admitted her to a sanitorium. His admission note exists. I've read it. It makes no claim of any cure. And it never even mentions any false pregnancy. And that entire business of reverse chronologic order. That, too, is conspicuously absent from that admission note.

So where did the case study come from? From whose pen? From whose fantasy? From whose theories?

And her dream. Of a snake. That represented her father's. . . . Obviously a fantasy on her part. All little girls have fantasies about their father's snakes. Especially those who told Freud that their fathers had sexually abused them. That obviously could not be true. Not in civilized Vienna. Decent people didn't even think of such acts. They had to be fantasies. But really whose fantasy was it? The girl's? The women's? Or their therapist's? Wasn't that really Freud's fantasy? Shaped by a failure to see reality? And how many women were mistreated by students of Freud because they confused Freud's fantasies with unfortunate reality?

Too damn many.

So, of course, Freud bashing is easy. Much of it, however, should be directed at his disciples. The Adlers, Reiks, and Alexanders of this world. For Freud made great contributions. Not just the unconscious and its role, but also the role of narrative in diagnosis, especially in psychiatry. Back to that again. Look at any nineteenth-century textbook on psychiatry. What do you see? Pictures. Pictures of the insane. Drawings of psychosis. Sketches of neurosis. Illustrations of craziness. A picture was worth a thousand words. People who had mental illness looked different. Not just those with melancholy. But the others also.

No more of that today. Not since Sigmund Freud. It's not what they look like that counts. It's what they say. It's their story. Words are all. A word is worth a thousand pictures. It's a truth no physician should ever forget.

But the disciples? Another issue. I've always felt that what Freud did to psychiatry was to remove it from the realm of science, testable science, and place it into the realm of faith. How did he do that? In the time-honored way. He taught disciples who then spread the word, his word, words that were true because he said them. If that isn't a religion, I don't know what is.

I have not mentioned Jung. Why? He deserves his own private condemnation. He out-Birkmayered Birkmayer.

Roger

December 19

Dear Rob,

Don't get angry at me. She doesn't work for me. She works for you. You are the one who hired her, not I. I wouldn't hire an antivivisectionist. Or is that term too old-fashioned for what she is? I'll admit it is a bit too stodgy and quaint, associated with images of suffragettes. Altogether too Victorian for most modern tastes. And too hard to spell. It's probably not even in my word processing program's dictionary. Now there is one of the true tragedies of modern life. Shakespeare never faced such dilemmas. In those days before Samuel Johnson's dictionary, how did you know if you had spelled a word correctly or not?

So you have a secretary, complete with word processor including a good dictionary, I hope, and this woman is an animal rights activist. And she read my letter to you. The one about Casablanca and the usual suspects. That's for the editor and the others, not you. Sorry. She read it and she was appalled.

So am I. And not merely by the cavalier invasion of our privacy. As I recall, my letter was addressed to you. Her name is not Rob, is it? For Robyn. Or Robin. Or Roberta.

I am appalled by her attitude, by her philosophy, and by her misinterpretation of the reality of what I wrote about.

How can she be opposed to all animal experimentation? Computers can't replace animals in all research. That's not how the game works. It's an antivivisectionist's fantasy. If we don't know what facts to put into the computer, the computer cannot give out the right answers. Especially not in relation to the effects and side effects of drugs. What does happen when you give drug X to an organism chronically? Is it safe? Is it effective? Or, like spearmint, does it lose effectiveness over time? Does it produce more side effects over time? Do we know enough to put all the facts into a computer? Hell, no. If we did, we wouldn't have to do the research. But we don't, so we have to. Would she take a drug whose safety in relationship to causing cancer was proven by a computer model? A breast implant, the safety of which relied on a computer program that couldn't possibly include all possible complications? Or what if she were pregnant—you do see pregnant women, I assume— would she refuse a Caesarean section because that procedure was first developed on poor, helpless experimental animals? Dogs, in that case, not guinea pigs.

Would she . . . but why go on? Logic is not the issue here. If it were, she would have attacked my research.

Let's take the worst case scenario. I told somebody to give something to some guinea pigs just to see what happened. That's what I was passing off as science. Something happened to those guinea pigs. They bounced up and down, just like kernels of popcorn. So we did it again. We so loved watching them bouncing and proving that what had been observed the first time was valid and reproducible. Science must always be reproducible. No place for coincidence. Nothing random. And besides, it was so much fun. Another batch of guinea pigs. More games in the ol' lab. And ran a dose correlation curve while we were at it.

And yet again and yet more fun. And this time we killed the poor guinea pigs. Need I tell you how? We stunned them and then removed their brains. Don't tell Rob that or she'll close us down. It was the best way to quickly obtain brains without changing their chemical makeup. And we did all of that just to measure some silly chemical or other. And we got results. Experiments work that way. They produce results. We scientists call that data.

But what did the data mean? I had no idea. But I did have the blood of those guinea pigs on my lab coat. Not my conscience, of that you can be damn certain.

Was I wrong to do what I did? No. It's called science. Gnosis. Knowledge. Research. Funded or not. The fact that these games with a few guinea pigs (which, by the way, were bred specifically for such games—or other games like cancer research) later explained a human disease is not the point. It merely makes the point.

Science is science. Good science, that is. Good science that asks a valid question. And the answer is significant. Sometimes even important. And no computer, so far, can tell which fact will be important some day. And which won't. All right. I'll get off my high horse.

Roger

P.S. Does she even know what a guinea pig looks like?

December 22

Dear Doctor Whose Name Is Being Withheld Out of Respect for His Family,
   NO.

Roger Kramer
Witness, 2nd Class

December 22

Dear Rob,
   I have no idea what to say. The card. His card. That card that doctor sent to me. You know which doctor. The protector of all good SS officers. And thus you know which postcard. His postcard. The postcard. The picture postcard. It was a Chagall. The picture on the postcard was a Chagall painting. Not a late Chagall parody of all other Chagalls. An early Chagall. A classic oil painting by Marc Chagall, the most Jewish of all Jewish artists. Not the most religious. Or the most observant. The *most* Jewish. It was classic early Chagall. A Chagall scene of a Jewish village. A shtetl scene. Out of Jewish Russia. Out of the pale of settlement. A scene of that world which is no more. The world destroyed by the SS. Why had he picked this artist? This style? This scene? Could it have been a random act? A coincidence? This is not literature. Was it for the irony?
   I threw it away. I have no more clever answers. Clever is not the answer.

Roger

December 27

Dear Rob,

I tried to write one other play. It was my Freud play. The actual title was *Anna O.* Although it was alternatively titled *Making Rounds.* That was a title that could have been out of Alan Ayckbourn. A real play on words. A double entendre, at least. More triple than double. It had to do with the story of Anna O. What was the real story? Who had lied? And to whom? The analogy to Ibsen was not lost on me.

Had Anna O. lied to Breuer? Lying to your therapist is not exactly a high crime. More like a misdemeanor. Patients do it all the time.

Had Breuer lied to himself? Self-delusion? Perhaps even more ubiquitous than lying to your therapist.

Had Breuer lied to Freud? A little boasting? Some clinical exaggeration. The clinical equivalent of a fish story.

Had Freud lied to us all?

Or had all of the above lied? For different reasons.

I had a great cast of characters. Most of them were obvious. What a great lineup: Freud. The judge of us all. Breuer. Anna O., at age sixteen. Bertha Pappenheim, at age fifty. Making them two characters gave me the opportunity to let her have two perspectives. And Arthur Schnitzler. He was my contribution to the story. If Shaffer can eliminate da Ponte, I can add Schnitzler. He takes out the writer, I put one in. He gets produced. There may be a message there. Somewhere.

So who was Arthur Schnitzler? Such is fame. Schnitzler was a Viennese physician and playwright. He is best remembered today as the creator of *La Ronde. Rounds.* That's the play in which each scene is a seduction scene and one character in each scene continues into the next scene with a new partner. A study in Viennese morals. Or the epidemiology of syphilis. Or AIDS. A companion piece to *The Blind Observer.* Schnitzler was one of the most famous Viennese writers of the first couple of decades of this century. And not because of *Rounds,* but because of his other plays. Plays that were widely produced. Some still are. And his short stories. And sketches.

So what did Schnitzler do? Not in real life, but in my play. In *Making Rounds.* Is the pun getting clearer? In my version, he helped Anna O. make up the stories she told to Breuer.

It was all very Brechtian. Each scene had a projected subtitle, taken from psychoanalysis. Subtitles like *Sublimation* and *Reaction*

Formation and *Transference*. And the scenes were not chronologically presented; they jumped around from the 1880s, when Breuer treated young Bertha, to the 1890s, when she became Anna O. in Breuer and Freud's book, to the 1920s, when Bertha and Freud and Breuer could all look back on what had happened. And so could Schnitzler. And the rest of us.

I integrated songs, pantomime, and even a trial scene based on a real trial that had taken place in Munich in the '20s. Schnitzler had been charged with writing pornography for *Rounds*. Since all of the sex acts took place when the lights were off and music was playing, the real trial revolved around the playing of pornographic music. In 1922. In Munich.

What an opportunity for a real burlesque. I cast Freud as the judge. Nice symbolism there. And Richard Strauss became a codefendant, since it was his music. It all, of course, had nothing to do with the play. The director never understood it. Or the actors. What did it have to do with character development? With the through line? Having never studied drama, I had no idea what the limits of a through line were. Nor what a through line was.

The scene was cut. Further progress. In my work in progress. To me it was pivotal. I haven't looked at it since that last reading.

Roger

Full manuscript available. Full-length play in two acts. Requirements: Four actors, two actresses, and a literate audience.
STRIKE THREE!

January

About once a month, until the age of 70, George Bernard Shaw suffered a devastating headache which lasted for a day. One afternoon, after recovering from an attack, he was introduced to Nansen and asked the famous Arctic explorer whether he had ever discovered a headache cure.

"No," said Nansen with a look of amazement.

"Have you ever tried to find a cure for headaches?"

"No."

"Well, that is a most astonishing thing!" exclaimed Shaw. "You have spent your life in trying to discover the North Pole, which nobody on earth cares tuppence about, and you have never attempted to discover a cure for a headache, which every living person is crying aloud for."

Harold L. Klawans
Newton's Madness

January 2

Dear Rob,

I should feel complimented by your remark, but Oliver Sacks and I are not exactly two peas in the same pod. Besides, why did you give your mother his complete works for Christmas? Why not mine? Other than the fact that his are all in print. A minor convenience. True, we are both neurologists. True, we are both neurologists who have a major interest in Parkinson's disease. Much more than an interest, a passionate dedication. A dedicated curiosity. And we both write real books. Not scientific treatises. But real books for real people. Trade publications for readers who read to read, not to carry out research. What a world of difference. We write for readers who read a book because they *want* to read it. Want to. Desire to. Think they'd like to. Not feel they must. That they have to. Not in that sense. Books to be read, perhaps even reread and savored, but not to be studied. Like old-fashioned novels, written to be read, not to be pored over by graduate students. Literature before Joyce, with a small l perhaps. And much of our writing has grown out of our experiences with our patients and our research on our patients. And we both read voraciously and have for years. And we both continue to write and to practice neurology. And the similarities do not end there.

Why do we write about disease? That's not the question, my friend. Our lives are surrounded by disease. We are enveloped by it, inundated by it. And we see what it does to patients, to their families, to their physicians, to ourselves. And how we all respond. Or don't. How could we do otherwise? Would Hemingway have written about an ambulance driver in the Great War had he not been one? Reread *A Farewell to Arms*. It's better than you recall.

The more intriguing question is why people read about disease. Why now? In such numbers? They never did before. It's not a natural subject. It's not part of classic literature. What Greek hero had a disease? Any disease? That bird devouring Prometheus's liver doesn't count. What Shakespearean hero? That lean and hungry look, as far as we know, did not come from consumption. In the nineteenth century, disease was in a novel for a reason, but never just to be a disease. The occurrence of disease as a result of risk factors never raised its statistical head. No competitive mortality here. Disease was a metaphor for something else. What? That varied from novel to novel. From opera to opera. Moral punishment, not endemic disease. A disease never stood for itself. Even

Hemingway couldn't get away from the symbolic use of disease. Why else did *Farewell* have to include death in childbirth? Certainly not to explore the medical or even the personal issues brought up by such experiences.

Now that has all changed. Why in the 1990s is the reader suddenly interested in disease?

Asked that way the answer is obvious. Or is it? It is to me. Because disease is a way of life now. And the way of death. Not hunger. Not war. Not any form of sudden death. Not even good old pestilence. But chronic disease. It has become our expected fate for the first time in our history. Dealing with disease is part of life. When Mozart died suddenly of an infection in his thirties, no one thought it was strange. People were expected to die suddenly of some unnamed cause. And life itself was the risk factor for such deaths. Now we expect to live long enough to suffer from some named disease. And most of us will get to fulfill that expectation. And many, more than once. More than one chronic illness. Cancer and kidney failure. Arthritis and. . . . You get the idea. So people read about disease. And we write about it. Not about the diseases as scientific issues but about patients with the diseases as humans coming to terms with human problems. Not symbolic problems, real ones. Cancer in your liver is not a metaphor for the decay of the inner city. On that you can bet.

But you could not call us close friends. Kindred spirits, absolutely. As far as I recall, we had never met before 1986. We were members of the same clubs who traveled in far different circles. We also read very different books. He can write about a patient with Parkinson's disease and relate that patient to James Joyce, D.H. Lawrence, Wittgenstein, Hermann Hesse, H.G. Wells. I'd be thinking about Hammett, Hemingway, Vonnegut. He quotes Kierkegaard; I quote Yogi Berra. Sure, our literary paths have crossed. I, too, have read T.S. Eliot. Who hasn't? But I distrust Eliot because of his anti-Semitism. Does Oliver? We never discussed him.

Also, we think about literature differently. And writing. And even neurology. The brain and its function, to Oliver, is often a philosophical issue. Or has philosophical implications. These issues are beyond me. I have never read Nietzsche. Nor Wittgenstein. And I never got all the way through *Ulysses*, or anything by Hesse.

I try to ask simple questions, questions that can be proven wrong by simple experiments. It's my training in research. No, that's not really right. It is how my mind works. That's why I did the kind of research I did. I had no idea how to approach the more complex issues. So each problem was conceived of as a set of simple, smaller issues. Issues that I could conceptualize. About which I could propose a hypothesis. And then set about disproving it. I may never have studied Karl Popper, but I know what he meant. The activity of dopamine at a dopamine receptor as a cause of a single jerk, not the organization of all dopamine neuronal systems neurons in relationship to the control of all human behavior. Oliver tries to understand the brain on a far different plane. That is the way his mind works. He can conceptualize philosophy, while all I can do is slug it out in the trenches. We see the world differently. Not antagonistically, but from complementary angles with far different approaches. Complementary approaches. At least I like to think so. But who remembers the guys who fought in the trenches? Did Hemingway? He only wrote about the officers.

David Garron remembers. He may be the only one. He still reads Siegfried Sassoon. And Owen. And the other poets of the trenches. Like Isaac Rosenberg. Yes. He, too, was an English poet of the Great War. One of the poets of the trenches. He is far less well known than Riley, Rilke, or Rimbaud. And not in the *World Book*.

In our own way Oliver and I have become friends. So when I was last in New York, I stopped by his office/apartment on 12th Street. Yes, I will now tell you that story. As a set piece. I call it *My Lunch with Oliver*. Here goes.

I followed Oliver as he stumbled down the five stairs toward the entrance to the Italian restaurant he had picked. There is another similarity between us, one that could serve as a major bond. I am certain that in grade school, or whatever that is called in London, he was also one of the last boys chosen to be on any team. It wouldn't have been for basketball or baseball, but for soccer or rugby. The exact sport made no difference. We were on our way to lunch, a meal neither of us needed but which we could not avoid. I had seen Oliver briefly at a "premiere" of *Awakenings* in Washington the previous week and told him that I would be in New York the next week and perhaps we could get together. He seemed to be enthusiastic. So I suggested lunch and he agreed and here we were.

He stood at the doorway, pursing his lips and stroking his overly full salt and pepper beard as if the strokes were needed to foster its further growth. Like talking to a plant or hugging a child. "They used to be harmless mannerisms, just little habits that I carried out, part of my unconscious personality. Now they all seem to be caricatures of Robin Williams," he said. "I no longer know if I do them unconsciously for the same reasons I always did them, or because I, for some unknown reason, need to copy his impression of me in order to be me."

He was both right and wrong and at the same time able to ponder the issue in his own quirky way. Robin Williams had obviously studied his subject very well. Far better than any of the movie critics realized.

We sat. We talked. The bread and butter arrived. We devoured it. We talked of many things. The movie. Obtaining more bread and butter. Originally, they had made him into a woman and Robert DeNiro had awakened to fall in love with her. That had been rewritten. And then Robin Williams had become Oliver Sacks, mannerisms and all.

"I am not a character," he protested.

"We all are," I consoled him.

We talked of the research on implants in treating Parkinson's disease, research I track far more closely than he does. I brought him up to date.

Our writing schedules. He went to the hospital only three days a week. He wrote on the other days. Jealousy. Not of his success. Of his available time.

Authors. Not Joyce. Not Lawrence. Not Hammett. Certainly not Hammett. Nor Ambler. But D.M. Thomas. Harry Mulisch. Julian Barnes. Poets. Auden. Cavafy. After all, I am not totally illiterate.

Abse. Dannie Abse. Welsh Jewish physician poet who lives, writes, and used to practice medicine in London. That was where Oliver had lived until he came to the United States to study neurology in the mid '60s. Did he know Dannie Abse? Were they friends?

"Yes."

I sat back. A story was coming. I could feel it generating. He pursed his lips. He stroked his beard. With a piece of bread, he wiped his plate clean. I followed suit. Imitation is the most sincere form of flattery.

"I was ten years old. It was during the war. Let's see. . . ," he paused. Another stroke. He picked up another piece of bread and studied it. His plate was clean. He put the piece of bread back down. "1944. No, '43. I'm certain it was '43. We went to one of his poetry readings."

At age ten. What was he doing at a poetry reading? He should have been playing baseball in the street, like I was. Or whatever kids played in the streets in London in 1943.

"I went with my mother. It was at the Cosmos Club. In Swiss Cottage. In London."

"He still lives near there," I chipped in.

"After the reading, we talked. I asked him about one of his poems."

At age ten.

"But we haven't spoken since. Not that I can recall. I think you would have to say that our friendship has lapsed."

Lapsed. 1943. Almost fifty years. Age ten!

"Do you know Dannie?" he asked me.

"Yes."

"How did you meet?"

"I wrote him a fan letter."

An approving nod.

"That was two years ago. I had never read any of his poems until then."

A disapproving stroke.

"I ran into a copy of his collected poems and wrote him a fan letter. We've become friends."

"Tsk."

"I was thumbing through the book. I saw his poem about Ezra Pound. The title got me angry. How could anyone write a poem in honor of that anti-Semitic SOB? I read it. Abse said everything I felt, everything that had to be said, far more eloquently than I could."

"He is a poet," Oliver reminded me.

"And I became a fan of his."

An approving nod combined with a twisting of a strand of his beard.

My story ends there. Our lunch didn't. Nor did our conversation. We continued to talk of things literary and neurologic. But most conversations are like most raw data in the laboratory—not worth studying. Much less publishing. If only most scientists were as self-critical as most authors. Authors realize that much of what they write is mere practice. Somehow scientists don't think that they, too, practice.

January 4

Dear Rob,

Were they all that in love with Alma? Was Gustav Mahler? Of course. Such a question. No one doubts it. Neither Gustav's biographers nor Alma herself in her own letters and memoirs. Alma completely dominated whatever life he had outside of music. That was why he was so crushed by her affair with Kokoschka that he sought out Freud. Those were the days of fashionable analysis. Especially in Vienna's intellectual Jewish community. So what about the others? Let's consider Kokoschka. He is the best starting place. It keeps her lovers in exact chronologic order, which makes far more sense than the other way around. Oscar K. is also easy to contemplate. He was not a truly great artist perhaps, but he did paint a few of the better paintings of this century. All right, that may be a bit of an exaggeration. A few damn good paintings. Ones that will last. Not a minor accomplishment. Oscar K. was also a man whose life spanned the eras of Emperor Franz Joseph and Ronald Reagan. Think about that. A single artist whose creative life spanned those two eras. Perhaps the world didn't change as much in those ninety plus years as we like to think that it did. But his art only obtained true intensity when Alma became a part of his life and thereby of his art. She had been the muse of much of Mahler's music. She became the muse and subject of some of O.K.'s art. That was shortly after Mahler died and before Alma chose Gropius over Kokoschka, architecture over painting, great tall buildings over flat surfaces—what would ol' Sigmund have made of that?

In 1913 Kokoschka painted a picture called *Two Nudes* or *The Lovers*. It's a picture of them; O.K. and Alma. They are the nudes. The lovers. Naked, and embracing like two waltzers. *Der Rosenkavalier* without clothes or music or that Straussian sophistication. And without von Hofmannsthal's words. We must never forget the words. But this is a painting. And such a painting. A painting of sheer lust. Lust in full color. Lust that needs no words. The next year came another work inspired by their affair. This one is called *The Knight Errant* and it is painted in far colder colors with strokes that are less bold, less powerful. The date was 1914. The war had started. The Great War. The War for Alma. Gropius was in the picture. Or rather Alma was in Gropius's picture and his bed. The Knight is lying down. He's exhausted. And there is Alma, a naked siren calling out to. . . . Take your pick.

O.K. went off to war—as an Imperial Dragoon. That must have been the last war with dragoons, Imperial or otherwise. He was shot in the trenches. And bayoneted too. Left for dead. And came home to Alma, who was now the wife of Gropius. So what did he do? What any other lust-filled returning Imperial Dragoon would do. He had a Munich doll-maker construct a life-size, soft, red-haired effigy of his beloved Alma, complete in every anatomic detail from breasts to vagina. All very gyne-cologic. Truly a man before his time. Had he been an entrepreneur, he might have marketed such dolls and made a fortune. But he was an artist. No mass-produced vulvas for O.K. He remained an artist. Perhaps our first conceptual artist. A surrealist before Tristam Tzara. Before Dada. Before André Breton gave leadership and a form of intellectuality to the surrealist movement. Certainly before Dali. O.K. lived with that doll. He shared his life with it. And his bed. But that was not all. I will not go into all the intimate details. He did, however, dress her up in fancy clothes and take her out for walks and to restaurants. In 1920 he painted *Self Portrait with Doll*, with the artist pointing at the doll's pudenda. Then he took the doll out one night with "some of the boys," got smashed, and they killed her—dumping her dead body into a garbage truck. Murder. Most foul.

Think of that doll. He was a man before his time. Did he love Alma? Was he obsessed by her? Does it matter? Or is it only the results that mat-ter? Not the dead doll. The pictures. O.K.'s pictures. *The Lovers. The Knight. The Self Portrait.* Three that will pass the test of time. Those three paintings are worth a thousand sessions on Freud's couch. And all the pain of O.K.'s lust for Alma. Did he realize that? How could he not have? Or would he have traded all three of them for a couple more hours in Alma's bed?

We'll never know. Unless we already do.

Owen died in the trenches where O.K had been left for dead. Only five of his poems had been published. So did Rosenberg. And Rupert Brooke. Sassoon, like O.K., recovered. Or didn't die. Instead he recreat-ed his life, becoming a fox-hunting man and wrote poetry that was far more eloquent, far more polished, with far greater elegance than his war poems. But without the intensity, or the immediacy. Or the bleak real-ism. O.K. had his Alma. Sassoon his trenches. Sassoon died in 1967. His life stretched from the Great War to the war in Viet Nam. Did he ever protest the latter? Even Clinton did that.

Roger

January 6

Dear Rob,

I spent yesterday afternoon in Northbrook. That's a suburb north of Chicago. It was all farmland when you interned here. Now it's quarter-million dollar houses, shopping centers, and some very fancy office buildings. I was in one of those. I was having my deposition taken. My very own deposition. It was round one of *Bloom vs. Kramer et al.* He was there. Martin Bloom. In person. The *real* Martin Bloom.

For someone who is dead, he looked pretty good. That is my opinion both as a physician and as an author/defendant. Not great, but pretty good. And short. A lot shorter than I remembered. In my memory, he was out on the pitching mound doing battle with the hated Yankees and standing tall. Six feet tall at least. They were all six foot tall warriors, the giants of my youth. He is closer to five seven or five eight.

And he's heavier than he was then, but who isn't? And his hair is gray. What color was it? Who knew? He had a White Sox hat permanently affixed to his head. The hat is gone, along with much of his hair. And he's probably put on about a pound a year—the national average. But it's been forty years. And traded in his Sox uniform for a gray business suit. He looked very much the prosperous insurance man that he is. He lives in Northbrook.

And so I sat opposite him. Opposite that left hand that had pitched not quite eighty-five innings, but had launched a single lawsuit. Not exactly a thousand ships.

We met in his lawyer's conference room. Altogether there were six of us. The lineup read like this:

For the defendant: Roger Kramer, right-handed witness and defendant. Randall Jackson, right-handed lawyer from the firm of Miksis, Smalley and Cavaretta, P.C. He was there, of course, to represent me. Joseph Tinker, left-handed lawyer. He was there representing Burt Shapiro of Sharp Books. Good ol' et al. Et al. was not there.

On the other side of the table, for the plaintiff we had: Martin Bloom, left-handed plaintiff. See previous description. William Evers, right-handed lawyer of Verban and Associates, representing Martin Bloom. Harriet Steinfeldt, right-handed lawyer, also of Verban and Associates, and also representing Martin Bloom. Bloom already had me outnumbered two to one. He'd never had the Yankees outnumbered. There was also one court reporter in the room. And if all works out poorly, I will be paying them all. Tinker, Evers, Steinfeldt. All lined up against me. What chance did I have?

Harriet Steinfeldt did the questioning. She started right in with the names. All the names in the whole damn book. Not all. In the prologue, I mentioned Tom Stoppard. Not the old Yankee pitcher, whose name I am withholding on the advice of my lawyer and my editor, even though I do not even have an editor for this yet, but Stoppard, the great British playwright. And the brilliant twentieth century philosopher Wittgenstein. But they aren't representing a philosopher. Or a playwright.

She started with the first story, "Did I Remove That Gallbladder?" It's the story of a real physician who had an attack of acute global amnesia, sudden memory loss, while operating on a patient. There he is in the operating room, *in media res*, and he can't remember what he's doing. What he's done. "Did I remove that gallbladder?" he asked over and over again.

A real story. Too good not to retell. I've seen dozens of patients with transient global amnesia, but had I not seen that patient, I would never have thought about telling about the disease by presenting an episode afflicting a surgeon in the middle of an operation. And people ask me if I am going to give up my practice. My books would suffer too much. It had to be written, like the story of my old friend, Walter Birkmayer, name unchanged.

I changed the surgeon's name. The first two words of the tale were his new name: Ken Keltner. Followed by an asterisk. With a note at the bottom of the page. "* All names have been changed for the purpose of this book." The surgeon, of altered name, had been rechristened Ken Keltner.

She read the first sentence, "Ken Keltner's name is not a household word." She left out the asterisk. Did I write that sentence?

I pleaded guilty.

Jackson said that we were willing to stipulate that I had written the entire book. After a prolonged conference, it was accepted that I had written each sentence in the book of which I was the author. The law at work.

Did I know who Ken Keltner was?

The surgeon I wrote about, I countered.

No, the source of the name.

"I'm unaware that there is only one Ken Keltner in the world," I said. "But why did you use that name?"

155

"It popped into my head."

"From where?"

"The lineup of the Cleveland Indians. 1948. He played third base. Had his greatest year in '48. He hit thirty-five home runs. His best game had been in '41. I don't remember that game. I wasn't even four years old at the time. He made two great plays that robbed Joe DiMaggio of hits and ended DiMaggio's hitting streak at fifty-six games. It's still in the record books. Fifty-six straight games. That may be why the name popped into my head."

She smiled. "How about the nurse, Joan Gordon?"

"What about her name?: I countered.

"Wasn't Joe Gordon the second baseman for those same 1948 Cleveland Indians? And didn't he have an outstanding season in '48, like Ken Keltner?"

"He did," I admitted grudgingly. Joe Gordon had spent most of his career with the Yankees.

"So, that is where the name came from?"

"I always thought Joe Gordon was a man. We may have to rewrite the history of baseball. And all those locker room encounters. Joan reminds me of Joan Crawford. And Gordon, of a brand of gin. And a Jewish third baseman—left fielder for the Giants. Sid Gordon. He also had a great year in '48. But not for the Cleveland Indians."

All I got for all that effort was a frown.

"Vera Bickford?" she asked.

Bickford was the patient on whose gallbladder the ex-third baseman had been operating. He'd also been a pitcher for the '48 Boston Braves. They had played the Indians in the '48 World Series. Spahn, Sain, and Bickford. Spahn's in the Hall of Fame. Sain ended up playing for the Yankees. Hence Bickford. He also appeared in *Sins*.

"Vera is our receptionist," I said.

"Bickford?"

"Charles Bickford, right-handed character actor."

She went on to another story. And another team. *The Man Who Would Save the World*. And John Lipon.

Shortstop. 1950 Detroit Tigers.

"Spontaneous generation." And Morton Cooper.

Pitcher. St. Louis Cardinals.

Walter Cooper?

Never heard of a Walter Cooper.

Didn't Morton have a brother Walker?

He did. Walker Cooper was great catcher. For the Cardinals and the Giants. In 1947 he hit. . . . So it went. And then we got to his story. The story of my Martin Bloom. Did I know there was a real Martin Bloom?

Yes.

Had I ever talked to him?

No. Asked his permission to use his name?

Why should I have done that?

He is probably the only Martin Bloom in the world. That's what she told me.

Did that give him exclusive rights to his name? Rights I might have to my name in any context. "Or Marshall Goldberg?" I asked her.

Who?

Halfback. Chicago Cardinals. Part of the dream backfield. And Jewish. His was the other name I'd debated using. Marshall Goldberg. Another childhood hero of mine. Were his rights the same as Martin Bloom's and vice versa?

No one answered me. They didn't have to. I was there to answer questions. Not to ask them, but my question was on the record.

Through it all, Martin Bloom glowered at me. As if he were on the mound staring down at Mickey Mantle. Snarled. Glowered. Relentlessly. And occasionally wrote down a note for Harriet Steinfeldt. Scribbled really with a gnarled arthritic left hand. The remnant of all those overhand curve balls.

My hero. Reduced to scribbling all but illegible scratches on a pad. My answers softened.

Harriet completed the survey. Rowe. Pitcher. Detroit Tigers. Gehringer. Second baseman. Detroit Tigers. A Hall of Famer. She was done.

It was Evers' turn. His job was to prove it was all my fault. That his client, Sharp Books, was an innocent victim of my wiles. More innocent even than the not-so-late Martin Bloom. His questions centered on some editorial phone calls. Calls that resulted in conversations between me as author and future defendant and a particular senior editor named Donovan. And one call in particular. The Donovan–Kramer call. Or was it a Kramer–Donovan call?

"Did you call Donovan?" he asked.

"No. I didn't even know he still worked for Sharp Books."

"Are you sure you didn't know that?"

"I'm sure. And I certainly didn't know he had anything to do with my book."

"And you tricked him?"

"I tricked nobody. It's all explained in the book. And I couldn't have called him. I didn't know his last name. I still don't."

"You knew his first name."

"Sure."

"Do you expect me to believe that you remember his first name but not his last name?"

"Of course."

"And why is that?"

"Because he used to pitch for the White Sox."

"Who?"

"Donovan."

"The editor for Sharp Books?"

"Of course not. The real Donovan. The one I remember. The name I remember. Dick Donovan. He was 16 and 6 in '55. Our best pitcher that year. The year I graduated from high school. He had a no-hitter going against the Yanks until the eighth inning. . . ."

No one seemed interested, so I stopped.

As always,

Roger

January 7

Dear Rob,

I know that this is my third letter in five days and that you have not even gotten around to answering my last half dozen letters, but I had the most absurd interview this afternoon and I had to tell somebody about it. The interview was about the practice of medicine today. That wasn't the subject. Just the subtext. About the realities. The inequalities. Not about all the acronyms. We never once mentioned DRGs or PPOs or HMOs or even Medicare. Medicare, I remind you, is completely egalitarian. It has reduced expertise to the level of mediocrity. A patient with Parkinson's disease comes to see me as a recognized authority on his disease. I must bill the same as any other neurologist. NO MORE. NO LESS. All doctors are equal. Who ever propagated that myth?

It all started last week when I got a telephone call from a reporter who was with *Chicago*. That's our city's answer to *The New Yorker* or *New York* magazine or whatever. It didn't exist back in the dark ages when you lived here. In any case, the reporter called me because he was doing an article for the magazine. It was going to be called "The Doctors' Doctors." The magazine had apparently taken a survey to find out which physicians the doctors in the Chicago area considered to be the very best. The survey had asked about a variety of specialties from allergy to vascular surgery and I'm sure included gynecology and obstetrics. To get their answers they had surveyed a large number of primary care physicians in the Chicago area (general physicians, family practitioners, internists, pediatricians, etc.) and asked them all the same question about each of these specialties. It was the precise question that they asked which intrigued me. What question would you ask? Who's the best plastic surgeon? Or to which rheumatologist do you send your patients? Simple. Straightforward. Well, Rob, they were far more clever than that. They wanted the best. The real best. So they asked the doctors whom they would choose to go to themselves or to send a member of their immediate family to see? To the editorial staff of *Chicago* that seemed to be the best way to get the information they needed; who really were the doctors' doctors? Fair enough. Maybe even brilliant enough to get reasonable information, to obtain honest data. And, after all, isn't honest data all you can ever really hope to get?

But, Rob, look at what they asked. Doesn't their very question imply a great deal about the way medicine is practiced in the United States and how patients individually and the public as a whole just accept it?

To make a long story a bit more concise than usual, the reporter described the survey and told me that I had been selected as one of the three neurologists to be listed in their doctors' doctor survey. One of the others was Barry Arnason. He's the Chairman of the Department of Neurology at the University of Chicago. His major interest is multiple sclerosis. The other was Nicholas Vick. He's the Chairman of Neurology at Evanston Hospital and one of the few neurologists whose main interest is the medical care of patients with brain tumors. I was thrilled. Make no bones about it. It's a nice honor. I'm in good company. And as long as they spell my name correctly, it will be good publicity. Maybe it will even help sell a few books.

But I was also disturbed. Aren't you? Think about it, Rob. Is that what we've come to? He told me he wanted to interview me and I agreed. Today was the interview. He spent an hour in my office asking me questions, all sorts of irrelevant questions, about my interests and accomplishments. When he was done, it was my turn. I asked him to tell me once again precisely what question they had asked the primary care physicians. I had to be certain I'd understood him.

He told me. "If you or a member of your family needed to see a neurologist, who would you pick?" Who, not whom. What do you expect from a journalist?

"Why," I asked, "didn't you merely ask them which neurologists they sent their patients to see?"

"That's obvious. We wanted to find out who were the best neurologists."

"I see. So you and your editors assumed that for most physicians only the best was good enough for them and their family, but for someone else the second best or third best or who knows, but clearly not the best, was good enough. Certainly for their patients."

"Right," he agreed, happy that I was educable enough to have understood their line of reasoning.

"Why is that?"

"What?" he replied, obviously caught off guard.

"Second best is not good enough for my patients. I always refer them to those physicians I think are the best, to the same ones I would go to myself, or send my wife or children to see. But I'm obviously in the minority. Physicians will send their wives and brothers and mothers, whatever, to see me or Barry Arnason or Nick Vick, but their patients can go see the neurologist next door. Doesn't that bother you?"

"No, not really. After all, there are some very good reasons for that."

"Name one!" I challenged him. "One that applies to anyone with a major medical problem."

"Convenience. You're halfway across the city. For patients from the suburbs, it could take them forty-five minutes to get here. Maybe more."

"The old Mercedes Benz issue," I commented.

He had no idea what I meant.

"Suppose you owned a Mercedes. It cost you thirty thousand dollars. Maybe more. I don't keep track of such things. It gets a flat. Okay, you take it into the nearest service station and get the tire fixed. No problem. But the motor is idling wrong. The transmission is acting up. Do you take it to the guys at the corner service station?" I waited for my answer.

"No," it finally came.

"You take it to the Mercedes dealer."

"So?" still somewhat puzzled.

"The Mercedes dealer is halfway across town." He was beginning to get the idea.

"You can always buy a new Mercedes. All you need is another forty grand or whatever it costs, but no patient can buy a new brain."

"Touché," he conceded.

"So the doctor who owns a Mercedes can drive forty-five minutes to have someone look at his car, but it's not convenient for his patient to go that far? Come on now. Neither of us actually believes that." And think how far he drives if he owns a Porsche. Or are you still into Corvettes?

"Why don't you run a second survey?" I asked. "In that one ask which neurologists they refer their own patients to and if they refer their patients to a different one, one who's not good enough to take care of their family, then why is second-rate care good enough for their patients?"

He didn't seem too interested. I'm sure they'll never run that survey. It probably would not sell newspapers. Or magazines. Or whatever.

But patients are catching on. Slowly but surely. They no longer rely on their family doctor the way they did. They call the experts. The United Parkinson Foundation, for instance. Or the Tourette Syndrome Association. That's who refers them to me. Maybe the doctors will catch on. I hope so.

Or do I? I'm backed up for two months as it is. How about you?

Medicare has, in its own way, caught on. In reverse. If a patient picks a recognized authority on Parkinson's disease and goes to see him on his own, without a referral from his doctor, Medicare will pay $55.00, but if his doctor refers him to some local yokel who isn't even board certified they'll pay $140.00. That's called progress. It's a great system, isn't it? Democracy at work.

Roger

161

January 9

Dear Rob,

Fred Gould called again, from Geneva. And he asked his same question once again. Had I changed my mind? I hadn't. The answer was still "no." Thank God, I have no other choice. We have a protocol, a protocol designed not just to protect our patients' rights, but to allow us to tell how well the patients do, to evaluate their clinical course as carefully and accurately as we can, and in so doing to evaluate how the procedure does, to test the implant procedure. To do that you need good follow-up of the patients. Of all the patients. Not just some, *ALL*. Follow-up is not something that Fred is good at. So I turned him down.

He asked me about the status of our program and I told him. So far we've done six implants. We took a break over Christmas. We'll get started again in a week or two. And the first four of the patients have now shown definite improvement. I told him that in December. I also told that to you. And everyone who was at our meeting. Those four patients have all continued to improve. They are better now than they were last month. For the other two, it's still too early to tell. See, I do include *ALL* the results.

"All four of them?" he asked me.

"All four of them," I told him.

"One hundred percent improved?"

"No!" I shouted back. "No one is one hundred percent improved. They all still need all their medicine."

"But," he countered, "one hundred percent of your patients are better."

Aren't statistics wonderful? "Yes, all four are better," I conceded. Four for four is one hundred percent. 1.000. A perfect batting average. Far better than my anemic .429. No, I haven't heard anything more from my agent. Thanks for thinking about it. If you were, that is. I was. But the patients are not cured. They still need all their medicines. They still have Parkinson's disease. They still have bad times every day.

"All four?" he asked again.

"All four," I again replied.

"One hundred percent then?"

"Yes," I admitted. I'm sure he understood what I really meant.

By the way, my paper got turned down. My paper on papers. My proposal. My editorial scheme. What ever shall I do? Guess.

Roger

Enclosures

Dear Dr. Kramer:
Your letter to the editor has been reviewed by two referees. While this letter is acceptable for publication, unfortunately it did not receive a high enough priority to allow us to publish it. I hope you understand that we receive many more acceptable letters etc. than we have space to publish. One of the editors was disturbed by your use of unsubstantiated hypothetical data. This is a scientific publication and as such must view the use of such nonscientifically generated data as highly suspect.

I thank you for allowing us to review your letter and hope that you will continue to submit papers to us for review in the future.

Sincerely,

Editor in Chief of
Journal

Rob: I wonder if *NEJM* has the same feel for data. I'm sure Garcia doesn't.

January 9

To the Editor of Journal Y
I am often asked to contrast the scientific and literary worlds....

January 12

Dear Rob,

I have finally made it to the big time. I've been asked to write a review for the Sunday *New York Times Book Review*, the literary world's answer to reviewing a grant for the NIH. Or reviewing an article for the *New England Journal*. The book was written by a psychologist from Vancouver named Stanley Coren. I've never met him, a prerequisite for reviewing his book, and I'm not particularly familiar with his research work. He is apparently a neuropsychologist, like David Garron. The book is called *The Left-Hander Syndrome*. Coren and his co-workers have been studying the issue of handedness for years. And they have come up with some fairly startling conclusions. And do I mean startling! According to Coren, left-handedness is never hereditary. Only right-handedness is. Man is always supposed to be right-handed. Woman, too. Not just much of the time or most of the time, but all of the time. Apparently God's original design was for one hundred percent right-handers. Sort of like one hundred percent acceptance of all scientific articles. Neurologically speaking, that means that the left hemisphere is always supposed to be dominant for handedness, just as it is for speech. In other words, all left-handedness is pathologic. It only occurs because something went wrong with the original plan, with the brain that should have been capable of following that blueprint. If that is true, then left-handedness is far more than a nuisance.

The book is more or less a summary of all the research that Doctor Coren, his associates, and many others have carried out over the past couple of decades in order to try to understand the meaning and implications of left-handedness. But it is also more than just a compilation of scientific data and the interpretation of such data, and here is where this book becomes worthwhile for the budding writer. Coren has told his story in a way that lets the reader in on his thinking as he tries to interpret his data, as he struggles to discover new hypotheses to explain the data, and scrambles to design further experiments to test each hypothesis. This is the real stuff of scientific investigation and it's all there to be chewed up and digested. Let me give you an example. It all started with his seemingly simple study of the frequency of left-handedness at different ages. At age ten, fifteen percent of the population is left-handed. At age thirty, the same condition exists. Nothing surprising there. After all, not having a scissors that fits your hand is not exactly a major health problem. But by age fifty, it drops down to six percent and by age eighty, there are virtually no left-handers left. None. Why is that? Where did all those left-handers go? Coren's analysis comes up with some pretty disturbing conclusions. The disappearance of left-handedness with aging is not due to slow adaptations of left-handers who over the years give up and start using scissors with their right hand. It is not a scientific "artifact" due to cultural influences that eighty years ago forced all left-handers to switch handedness so that the "decrease" in handedness is merely an expression of changing societal acceptance of left-handedness. Left-handers seem to disappear because they die off. Their life expectancy is less than that of those whose hands fit those scissors. Not just because of accidents caused by life in an alien, right-handed world, but because left-handedness carries with it an increased liability to certain diseases.

By the way, you are not left-handed, are you?

Now all I have to do is expand my letter to you and my book review is done. Two birds with one stone. I knew these letters would come in useful, even if no one ever publishes them. What a thought!

You do, I assume, read the *New York Times Book Review*. Or, if not you, your mother.

Roger

January 17

Dear Rob,

Since when did you start reading *Neurology*? Isn't that a bit out of your field? I certainly don't read any of your journals. Or is it your mother who subscribes to *Neurology*, right along with the *Chicago Sun Times*, and then sends you the articles she thinks would be of interest to you? An interesting range of reading material that, the *Chicago Sun Times* and *Neurology*. Throw in *Vanity Fair* and *Screw* and she'll have all the bases covered.

At least you understood the title, *Pyramid Sale in the Bucket Shop*. Most of the members of the PSG didn't. I do know what a pyramid scheme is, I'm not that naive. Hell, I've even fallen for such schemes. Not monetary ones. The usual letters and all that. But I had no idea what a bucket shop was. I thought it was a place where they made buckets. Or sold them. Or both. Not someplace where the primary goal was to swindle investors by various illegal or unethical practices.

What did we do that was illegal? What did we do that was unethical? We tried to test a hypothesis. A hypothesis carefully designed to be testable. Does Eldepryl slow the progression of Parkinson's disease? A good, simple, important hypothesis. Scientifically rigorous. And clinically significant. We designed the best experiment we could to test that hypothesis. A couple of dozen of us spent over a year working on the design. Not me. At least I didn't do much of the substantive work. I helped primarily by raising some of the money to support all the preliminary work and by giving some advice and a bit of sage critique, as becomes a senior investigator. Others did the work. And it involved a lot of work. First there was the design itself, then the power analysis. How many patients did we need to study? That is not a simple question. You have to decide on the variability of your groups, the degree of difference, and then the statistician gives you the answer. Eight hundred! Double blind, of course. Placebo control. And then there was the selection of the scales to be used. We didn't invent our own. Then the work to verify and validate these scales to guarantee interrater reliability. Did we all see the same symptom in the same way? Then came writing the formal grant itself. The organization of the thirty centers. The coordination of those centers and the data collection. The interpretation of the data, all carefully designed prior to collecting the data. Of course, we were concerned that Eldepryl might have had a mild therapeutic effect and that the therapeutic effect might have been responsible for our result, so that it only seemed as if we had actually slowed the progression of the disease, but we really hadn't. We'd just made those patients feel a little better. That would mean that the reason the patients didn't get worse was that they were being treated with an active drug, not that their disease was not progressing.

We knew that was possible. That's why we designed the study the way we did. But our results were so significant, so striking, and the so-called therapeutic effect so minimal, that the latter could not cause the former. At least that's what our biostatistician told us. With a reasonable degree of scientific reliability.

So what did William Landau call us? A pyramid sale in the bucket shop. Practitioners of neuromythology! And, yes, I write science. I also write myths. I know the difference between the two.

And he accuses us of newspeak. You may have been right to read Orwell. At least we did nothing that was Kafkaesque. And then to say our study was an example of the Patty Hearst phenomenon, that some scientific version of the Symbionese Liberation Army seemed to have brainwashed us.

He might be right about our data analysis. I'm not a biostatistician. Some of the arguments he raised about data interpretation are far beyond my level of competence. He could be right about those. It might all be nothing; just a mild beneficial effect. *Might* I said. I doubt if he is right. We had a lot of good people working on this.

But he is also wrong. We used no newspeak. We invented no new form of double-talk. And we perpetrated no intentional pyramid scheme. It was not a bucket shop. We were trying to answer a scientific question as best we could. Scientists have been wrong before. Damn good ones. And will be again. We may have created a myth but not intentionally.

I guess you should sell any Mylan you bought. And read more Orwell.

Roger

January 22

Dear Rob,

You're absolutely right; I would love to become a literary groupie. I would be if I could; but I can't. There ain't no group.

Is it just my own private fantasy? To have my own Parisian style moveable feast right here in Chicago. To have a group of fellow artists, fellow writers, especially writers, to live, work, breath, eat, drink, and fight with. Argue, that is, not actually fight as in boxing. I am not Ernest Hemingway. But to be able to drink Pernod with Hemingway. Figuratively. Literally. Except it wouldn't be Pernod. I tried Pernod once. It all but made me nauseous. And it wouldn't be with Hemingway.

Writing is a lonely craft. And writing without anyone else who writes is both lonely and isolated. And those who are not involved in the craft or a similar craft cannot change that sense of isolation.

David helps. His toe is better, by the way, in case you were wondering. And his physician is even talking to him. Barely.

Perhaps I'm too spoiled by medicine. Perhaps my expectations are all wrong. No one wins a Nobel Prize in medicine in isolation. No, I do not expect to win a Nobel Prize in medicine. It's in physiology and medicine officially. Nor in literature. Certainly not. But I know Nobel laureates in physiology and medicine. I've been to meetings with them. I've been on programs with them. We've served on panels together, worked together. That's the way the field of medical research is organized.

In '71 I was three years out of my residency, I was invited to participate in a meeting of the World Federation of Neurology Research Group on Huntington's chorea. There were a total of perhaps three dozen people involved in that group. There I was, still wet behind the ears, and rubbing shoulders with the neurologic superstars. Stars like Sigwald Refsum.

Who was he? The leading Scandinavian neurologist of this century. He discovered his own disease. A world expert on hereditary neurologic diseases. He died last year.

My Refsum story. I have more than one. I'll only tell one. It's about a pneumoencephalogram. A pneumo: we used to do pneumos regularly. They've been part of our history since the invention of the CAT scan. A pneumo was done by doing a spinal tap and replacing the spinal fluid with air. After the air got up to the brain, you took x-rays to get an outline of where the air was, an outline of the shape of the cavities of the brain. It was primitive. And painful. Sort of medicine à la Fu Manchu. Well, in Refsum's book on the neurologic examination, he published a normal pneumo. Or, more correctly, the films of a patient with a normal pneumo.

What's the big deal about that? I'll tell you. It's Quisling's pneumo. Quisling was the Norwegian Prime Minister under the Nazis in World War Two. A true Nazi collaborator. Worse than Birkmayer. Or Jung. When the war was over, the Norwegians tried Quisling for collaboration and along the way did a pneumo to make certain there was no neurologic basis for his apparent behavior. There wasn't. The pneumo was normal. Perfectly normal. *The* normal pneumo. Just look in Refsum's book. It's there.

Then they shot Quisling. Reversing the original process. The pneumo was a by-product of the Great War. A soldier was shot in the head. An X-ray showed air outlining his brain. And he was alive and awake. Before that no one knew that could be done. That air inside the brain was safe. From that observation, it was a short step to doing pneumos. Short but significant. The Norwegians reversed it all. Air first, then the bullet.

That's my Refsum story. Or rather one of them. You see, we became both friends and collaborators after that meeting.

Who else was at that meeting with a story to tell me?

MacDonald Critchley. President of the World Federation of Neurology. The world's expert on the parietal lobes of the brain.

We, too, became friends. He told me the story of a patient of his, a German Jew. Born and bred in the Fatherland as a reformed, integrated, totally assimilated Jew who spoke nothing but German. He had married in the twenties, had two children, was active in the German Communist party. His wife, who wasn't Jewish, was more active. Come 1933, he got out. His wife didn't. His kids didn't. He escaped into France. He lived in hiding throughout the entire war with a French family and their daughter. When he learned that his wife and children were dead, he married the French girl. They had a child. The three of them spoke only French together. That one child, a girl, was the delight of his life.

His French wife died in 1949 and he moved to England. There were some cousins living there. He learned English and went into business as a toy manufacturer. He was free and accepted for the first time in his life and after a few years became successful and rich. When he was sixty he retired and traveled extensively. He took a trip to Israel and for the first time really became a Jew. At age sixty-two he learned Hebrew.

For the next four years he spent six months in Jerusalem and six months in London with his daughter. He went to synagogue each day. Then at age sixty-six he had a stroke, and it involved his speech. Aphasia. Now what language was he left with? Let's look at the possibilities.

German? The language he was born with and raised with. His only language until he was thirty years of age. The language he'd married in and had two children in.

French? The language of escape. The language of his second marriage. The language of his daughter. They always spoke French together.

English? The language of freedom and of success of the last fifteen or so years before his stroke.

Hebrew? A latecomer. Learned only at age sixty-two.

Which one?

That's right. Hebrew. Not German. Not French. Not English. Hebrew. Hebrew—but why? I'm not sure I know, but Critchley thought it had to do with the meaning of the language. The emotional meaning to the patient. That language that has the greatest meaning—emotional meaning—has the widest representation in the brain and is most likely to be spared. Hebrew meant the most, was the most important language, so it was the one that was least affected. For years he lived in Jerusalem and each day walked to the Wall. So much for Critchley's story.

That's the kind of story that might well appeal to Oliver. I'm sure he'd be able to interpret it far better than I. To integrate it into a deeper understanding of the brain. Perhaps I'll send him a copy of these letters. Oliver, by the way, is not the first famous physician-writer named Oliver. Oliver St. John Gogarty has that honor. He was, you recall, both a physician and a poet. A friend of James Joyce. Joyce satirized him in *Ulysses* as Buck Mulligan. End of friendship. Perhaps I won't send these letters to Oliver.

So in medicine, I'm spoiled. I not only work in a medical school with a research milieu, I know and break bread with the best. And I always have. Unless the elite share their ideas, science would not grow in the way it does. Medicine can not thrive in isolation. I want that same sense of sharing in my other life.

But what about Albert Schweitzer, you ask? I knew you would think of him. Working alone. In a small clinic in the middle of the Congo. It's Gambia today, I think. Bringing modern medicine to Africa. And he won the Nobel Prize.

Wrong. On both counts. He never brought modern medicine to anyone. Battlefield surgery, perhaps very good field surgery, but not real modern medicine. No one man could do that. Even then. And he won his Nobel Prize in peace, not medicine.

So I dream of having Pernods with Hemingway. And end up having a rare lunch with Oliver. And talking Sassoon with David. And Alma Mahler.

Roger

February

"It was here," Paul told them, "that the Crusaders spent their first Sunday in Jerusalem. Right here on the top of the Mount of Olives.

"Here these great nobles from France, England, Italy, and Germany found a Christian hermit, an old man, who lived in a cave on the Mount of Olives undisturbed by the Muslims below. This one man blessed them and prophesied that if they would attack Jerusalem right then from right there, the attack would succeed. It would be God's will. The knights mounted their horses, charged down into Kidron Valley, and then attacked the eastern wall of Jerusalem."

"What happened, Dad?" Joshua asked.

"Guess."

"The Crusaders won."

"No. They got creamed. A prophetic blessing is no substitute for an adequate battle plan."

Harold L. Klawans
The Jerusalem Code

February 2

Dear Rob,

My first paper? God, that seems like it was such a long time ago. More like ancient history than part of my own career, yet it occurred a mere twenty-five years ago. It concerned a patient whom I never met until after his autopsy, not exactly a formal introduction. A modern variant of the meeting between the Inquisition and Garcia d'Orta, but the other way around. I tried to illuminate his life, not eradicate it. There is a difference, I think.

I was a second-year neurology resident doing six months of neuropathology with Orville Bailey. This patient's brain was one of the numerous brains we cut during one of our weekly brain cutting sessions. As you probably remember, the central nervous system is not actually examined during a routine autopsy. It's removed during the autopsy proper and put in formaldehyde to fix it. And then a week or so later it's preserved well enough to be studied. That was how I met the patient. I showed up a week after his autopsy in order to assist in the cutting of all of the fixed brains. This particular patient's brain just happened to be ready to be cut. And so was his spinal cord. That was where his disease process was located.

He had a peculiar form of syringomyelia. I know that to you, as a gynecologist, all forms of syringomyelia must seem peculiar. They are all admittedly rare, these tube-like cavities in the spinal cord. That's what syrinx means—a tube. Almost all of them are congenital problems that begin in the neck. Not so this man's. His began in the lower part of his back and not because of some congenital abnormality of his spinal cord. Far from it. He'd been in an accident and his spinal cord had been crushed. He'd recovered some function, but been left paralyzed in both legs. Then years later he'd developed progressive neurologic problems that showed that something was wrong with his spinal cord above the level of his old injury. But what exactly was the problem? No one knew. Until he died and Orville looked at his spinal cord and found a tube coming right out of his old crush injury. That was something that Orville had never seen before. And if he hadn't seen it, I was pretty sure no one else had, but that was mere conjecture on my part. Orville was also fairly certain he'd never even read about such a case. I was willing to take his word for that. He wasn't. And there was only one way to be certain. So I was sent off to the library to read the world's literature on the neurologic complications of spinal cord injuries.

That was my first attempt to review the medical literature, completely, exhaustively. Not out of curiosity, but to see if what we'd observed was something new or something others had seen before, and, almost as important, to me at least, did the literature (THE LITERATURE, I've always loved the sound of that short phrase) explain our observation and, if not, would publishing our observation be a valid contribution to that literature? A contribution to THE LITERATURE. Not *Heart of Darkness*. Not even *The Murders in the Rue Morgue*. But a real contribution.

It was exciting. It was heady. Wandering around the stacks of the library, pulling out old journals. Those were the days before computerized searches and Xerox copies supplied by anonymous copy machines of just the exact pages you needed to read.

But how could I know what I really wanted? The 1915 *British Medical Journal*, the British answer to *JAMA*. Or vice versa. It had the classic articles on spinal cord injury by Gordon Holmes, one of the leading clinical neurologists of the first half of this century. And, as far as I know, no relation to Sherlock. Watson mentions brother Mycroft but no cousin Gordon. But that one bound volume of journals had so much else in it. So many articles that had nothing to do with neurology, much less syringomyelia. The succeeding article was a discussion of the history of eyeglasses. An anonymously derived Xerox copy would never have included that article. I read every word of it. I now had two subjects I wanted to devour completely.

The Holmes article helped. Holmes had been in the Great War. He was one of those doctors to whom Hemingway could have delivered the wounded soldiers. Except he worked on a different front, France, not Italy. So they probably never met. Did Holmes meet Sassoon? Or Owen? Holmes treated injured soldiers and after they died he did autopsies and looked at the spinal cords of those who had had spinal injuries. Medical science at work. Learning from the destroyed bodies of the friends and compatriots of Sassoon and Owen. And Rosenberg. We mustn't forget him. It was a different sort of legacy of that slaughter of innocents. After reading Holmes' article, I understood the spinal cord better. It is much like a long, thin tube of toothpaste, and in a crush injury the cord acts just like toothpaste in a tube does when the tube is suddenly crushed. The contents of the tube get squeezed in two different directions. The soft material that is the center of the cord is squeezed into the normal uncrushed cord above it. Later these displaced tissues die, leaving a cyst. Holmes described that. A small cyst caused by a crush injury of the spinal cord. That had to have been what had originally happened in our patient and then the cyst grew slowly over the years. Cysts tend to do that.

Had that ever happened before? Holmes was silent on that question. Or since Holmes, but before our case? My case? If Burt Shapiro can change possessive pronouns, so can I. And I first met him ten years later.

Back to the stacks. More rummaging. More dust. More sidetracks. More on eyeglasses. Did they really somehow find their way to our noses without our knowing where or when or how? Or who? And then I found the missing link. Holmes had studied acute crush injuries in British soldiers injured during World War One. Most such patients died. Not just the ones he studied, but most of the others too. In World War Two, most of them survived. Many ended up in spinal cord units of VA hospitals. And years later a few of them had developed a progressive spinal cord syndrome, just as my patient had. [Note the transition.] A Canadian neurologist named Barnett had described some cases just the year before. He thought they might have syringomyelia, but he had no proof.

Well, I had the proof. Or, rather, Orville did. So I told Dr. Bailey what I had learned. He listened. "Just what I thought, no one else has seen it."

"Barnett," I began. . . .

"No one has seen it. He's seen patients he thinks might have this specific variety of syringomyelia, but no one else has really seen it. You will write it up for publication."

You will. Not you might. Or you could. Or should. Will. So I did, and that became my first publication, but not without a few tribulations. Once the paper was finished and Orville had approved it, I submitted it to *Neurology*. They rejected it. Why? The editor, Russell De Jong, felt that the concept that trauma could cause syringomyelia was too controversial in a medical-legal sense for him to publish such a revolutionary notion based on just one case.

Second choice? A British journal. *Neurology, Neurosurgery, and Psychiatry*. Why? Medical-legal issues were less touchy in the U.K. and Gordon Holmes had once been the editor. Another rejection. Why? Their editor, John Walton, felt that the paper added nothing new. Everybody knew that trauma could cause syringomyelia. That had been proven long ago.

Eventually my paper found a home. And recognition. I was thrilled. I was batting 1.000. Little did I know then that everybody hit 1.000. Five years later in his book *Syringomyelia*, Barnett borrowed my slides and used them to show the pathology of a syrinx caused by trauma since it was still the only proven instance in THE LITERATURE.

Around the time that book was published, at one of those noisy, over-crowded receptions hosted by the American Academy of Neurology, I found myself in a small group including Russell De Jong, John Walton (by then Sir John Walton), and H.J.M. Barnett. Some coincidence, that. It was also too good an opportunity to let pass, so I didn't. I now wish I had. I started off by discussing "our" case with Barnett.

"Why," he asked with some prompting, "had it been published in such an obscure journal?"

"*Neurology* turned it down," I said.

"Why?" he asked turning to the editor.

Dr. De Jong could not remember.

I could and I did. "But so did the *Journal of Neurology, Neurosurgery, and Psychiatry*," I added.

"John?" Barnett said, quizzically.

Sir John could not remember. I could and I did. Barnett loved it. Two editors having turned down the same paper for opposite and equally invalid reasons. Mine had been the first proven case.

I loved it, too. I don't anymore. Russell De Jong had not rejected my paper personally. One of his sub-editors had. Same for John Walton. It hadn't been their choice, their decision. Had they even read my paper? Unlikely. The job of the editor-in-chief is to delegate authority and keep everything running smoothly. Not to read every rejected article.

I know that now. And I wish I hadn't embarrassed them both. And myself.

Roger

175

February 4

Dear Rob,

The Dahmer case has made me angry. I'm sure I don't have to explain who Dahmer is. That in and of itself may well be a commentary on the state of our civilization. We all know Dahmer. Do we know who won the Nobel Prize for literature last year? Or this year? It sure as hell wasn't Dahmer. Or Amy Fisher. Dahmer was too busy becoming America's most recent bizarre serial killer, storing his victims' body parts in his deep freeze and then eating them. Pouring acid into their brains to convert them into love slaves. So his is a name Americans know. Like the Son of Sam. Not Rilke. Nor Kokoschka. Nor even Mahler. Gustav or Alma. I'd settle for either one. The Dahmer case has gotten an inordinate amount of coverage here. Milwaukee is just a stone's throw north of here. Some of his victims were from Chicago. The trial is being broadcast live. A regular circus. It's not the atmosphere that has gotten to me. Nor his crimes. Nor what he did to those poor guys. Things like that happen. So he poured acid into guys' brains to make them love slaves. And kept their bodies. And ate parts of them. Stored their heads in his freezer. Etc. Etc. Insanity like that has always been with us. It always will be. That's not what aggravates me. It may appall me, but much of human behavior does that. Dahmer's not the real perversion in this case.

There was a study once by somebody at the National Institute of Mental Health. It was back in the early '70s. That was the heyday of the NIMH. This study was done by either Bunney or Goodwin, I think. No matter. The study itself didn't add very much to our understanding of affective disorders or change our way of treating the patients, nor unfortunately did it change how we think about disease. The study was primarily the study of some new anti-manic drug. I don't remember which drug. It was also a study of how to carry out such studies, a sort of research on research. They studied the various scales used by psychiatric investigators when studying mania. Back to the problem of scales again. Are we measuring what we think we are measuring? And are we measuring it accurately? Mania is more like Parkinson's disease than blood pressure. How do you measure mania? What scale do you use? Is the scale accurate? Do different people see a single patient and rate him the same way on the scale—is there interrater reliability? They studied all of the available scales and trained everyone in the use of the scales; nurses, social workers, psychiatrists, the whole team including the nurses aides. They were almost ready for the study. They added one more scale—but gave no special training on this scale and no explanation. It was called the craziness scale. Each rater would rank how crazy the patient was that day on a scale of zero to ten. Zero meant not crazy at all. Not "normal," just not crazy. Ten meant crazier than a bedbug. Or a loon. Or whatever. As crazy as possible.

On to the study and the results. The drug may or may not have worked. No matter, we have lots of drugs that work a little bit. The craziness scale did. Of all the scales they used, it had the highest degree of interrater reliability. Higher than all the fancier scales with all their built-in guidelines and definitions and training. The craziness scale was the best.

Why? Because we all know what craziness is. We each have a common sense definition, a practical unsophisticated scale unfettered by jargon, unprejudiced by scientific theory. Crazy is as crazy does. And we all can recognize that craziness and rate it—reliably. We recognize bats-in-the-belfry. Any belfry. Any species of bat. And can tell how many bats are there. With very good reliability. Interrater reliability.

Or do we?

Look at what is going on in Milwaukee. It's a perversion. A perversion with a very low level of interrater reliability. Fifty percent agreement. One half. No better than random chance. But nothing is random. Nothing at all. The psychiatrists working for the state of Wisconsin say that Dahmer is sane. We all know that people who pour acid into the brains of sex partners are really rational, sane human beings. And necrophilia? Everyone could be into that. And who knows what your neighbors are storing in their deep freezers? To say nothing of cannibalism. The psychiatrists for the defense say he's insane. Crazy. A ten on any scale. If not greater. So much for interrater reliability.

Look at the question. If Dahmer doesn't fulfill every single common sense definition of insanity, then who the hell does? No sane man could do what he has done. On a scale of zero to ten, he must be a twenty. So why would the state waste money trying to prove that he is sane? He can't be. He isn't. Trying to play games with some technical legal definition of insanity is itself a form of controlled lunacy. Is that what our system of justice is all about?

So why? So they can prosecute him as a murderer. Because if he's crazy, he goes to a state mental institution—not exactly a trip to Hawaii. And each six months he can petition for release. He could be out in six months doing his crazy thing again. As if any psychiatrist would ever say he's cured. No longer crazy. He'd always be at least a ten. Look at what he's done.

If his being crazy means he goes into a mental institution and that is frustrating—change the law. Don't pervert psychiatry. Dahmer is INSANE. He's crazy. He'll always be crazy. Calling him sane is no better than what the Russians did. They called sane people crazy in order to incarcerate them as punishment for what they had done. Major crimes. Like wanting to leave Russia, the worker's paradise. For refusing to love communism. True insanity, that. And we call Dahmer sane in order to incarcerate him for what he's done.

Is what we might be doing any different from what they did? Any better? It may be worse. We believe what we are doing is morally and ethically correct. And legal. The Russians didn't care. They had no such pretensions.

In its own way, the defense is equally perverted. Their psychiatrists tell us that we should study Dahmer. We can't miss the opportunity. A case study. The case study from hell.

How? Where would we start? Who knows? Not the psychiatrists, that's for sure. They can't even agree that he's crazy. And if he's not, what's to study?

Roger

February 6

Dear Rob,

Did I know that André Breton was a physician? What a question! One of his poems even contains a description of the treatment of angina. He was much enamored of Freud and psychoanalysis. Freud, via Breton, had a major influence on surrealism. So did Rimbaud. Did you get to him yet? Later Breton became even more enamored with communism. Pure communism. He and Leon Trotsky co-founded the Independent Federation of Revolutionary Art. In 1938, before Stalin had Trotsky assassinated. True, they would have had trouble co-founding it afterwards. Breton spent the war years in the United States and remained the chief promoter of surrealism and himself until he died in 1966.

But not all physician-writers were important. Or heroic. Not even all French physician-writers. Take Louis-Ferdinand Céline for instance. Céline was a physician. And he, too, was an important writer. He's often credited as one of the founders of modern French literature. Sort of a French Ring Lardner who freed French literature from the shackles of "good writing." He, too, was initially attracted to communism and, like Orwell, became disillusioned. Unlike Breton, he remained in France throughout the war and after it was over he was convicted of having been a Nazi collaborator. Neither of his two careers was an excuse for such behavior.

I saw a patient named Gonzales today. He's been a patient of mine for about eight years. Mexican-American. He's had Parkinson's for about a dozen years. He's quite disabled. He is still a rather young man, in his early fifties. We've tried everything. All the experimental drugs. I can't remember when he was last able to work. His wife works for the Chicago Board of Education. She's a cook in one of the high school cafeterias. She supports them both. Since she works, they always come in late in the afternoon. She always comes in with him. I sometimes think they were interested in all those experimental protocols because the medications are free and so are all the blood tests and the doctors' visits.

I hadn't seen them in four months. He looked better than he'd been in a couple of years. I checked his chart. I hadn't given him anything new. I hadn't even changed his dosages. Same old medication, yet he was walking better and his voice was stronger.

"What happened?" I asked.

He'd been to Mexico City and seen Garcia.

"Did he do an implant?" I asked. Once informed, I looked and could see the telltale scars on his scalp. He'd obviously undergone a craniotomy. Always the astute observer.

"No," I was told.

"No?" I could see the scars.

"He charges too much. Too much dollars."

I frowned.

"From me, he wanted forty thousand dollars. I don't have that kind of money. I went instead to Monterrey. My wife, she has family there. Her brothers. There is this neurosurgeon there. He's not a big man. Not famous. This neurosurgeon he studied with Garcia. He operated me for five thousand dollars. That much dollars we had. And I am better, no?"

"You are better, yes," I agreed. "Not cured, but better."

He was still on all his medications, but they were more effective. He was improved, much like our own patients. He has more "on" time. Less "off" time. His "offs" are not as off. He won't go back to work, but his life is a lot better. There is still one unanswered question—how long will it last?

What do we charge our patients? Insurance only. That's it. We, the neurologists and the neurosurgeons and even the hospital, are taking nothing from the patients themselves. They shouldn't have to pay for our research.

Roger

All right. I admit it. I didn't know that Breton was a physician.

February 10

Dear Rob,

What a morning! I went to the Chicago Sports Memorabilia Show. Sports nostalgia packaged to sell within any price range you can afford. I've never been into memorabilia. Nostalgia, yes. But nostalgia based on memories, or thought, not on objects.

They had it all. Old White Sox uniforms. Programs. Tickets. Autographed baseballs. Hats. Bats. Everything but jock straps. And, of course, baseball cards. I used to collect them. Who didn't? I even had Mickey Mantle's rookie card. Who didn't? My mother gave them away. Whose didn't? It was part of their job description. And it's a good thing that she did. Today that card is worth thousands. If my mother hadn't thrown it away and if every other mother hadn't, it'd only be worth five bucks.

I went looking for one thing and one thing only. Martin Bloom memorabilia. A picture of Martin. Marvelous Marty. A baseball card of my one-time hero, Martin Bloom. At each booth I asked, "Any cards of Martin Bloom?"

"Who?" the first proprietor asked me.

I explained.

"Never heard of him. Does he even have a card?"

I took the man's business card. Why? He could become an expert witness. An expert on the commercial value of Martin Bloom's reputation and renown.

Within an hour I had pursued the same question at over a dozen booths with almost twenty sales people, all experts on baseball memorabilia. The answer remained the same: "Who? Never heard of him." And I kept on collecting business cards. At the last booth, I finally found one. A Martin Bloom card! It was printed in 1951. A Bowman card. It existed. Martin existed. I knew that. He's suing me. He must have existed. He has to exist. He can't be dead.

1951 was his big year.

I bought the card and am sending a copy to you. I also bought three baseballs, three autographed baseballs, one autograph per ball. Luke Appling, Chico Carrasquel, and Luis Apparicio. Forty years of great shortstops.

And . . . memorabilia is contagious.

I almost bought a Cub card. A card of a Cub. Can you believe that? The only card of a Cub player ever of literary significance, Eddie Waitkus of not-so-sainted memory. We have Shoeless Joe Jackson. And the rest of the Black Sox. And Monty Stratton, who shot off his legs and then tried to make a comeback. James Stewart played him in the movie. And the rookie who wrote those letters in Ring Lardner's *You Know Me, Al*. He played for the White Sox.

And all the Cubs have is Eddie Waitkus, who made his mark as a member of the Philadelphia Phillies. Such is fame.

Roger

***

Martin Bloom
Pitcher, Chicago White Sox
1951 Bowman

Editor's Note. This card remains under copyright and cannot be reproduced without permission. We were unable to obtain permission. Our request was returned marked, "Deceased—Return to Sender."

February 11

Dear Rob,

They found Dahmer sane. The American judicial system at work. They heard all the witnesses. Half the psychiatrists said he was sane. Half said he was insane. Then the jury met to reach their decision. And reach it they did. The jury voted 10-2. By an overwhelming majority they decided that this serial sexually aberrant killer was SANE. NOT CRAZY. SANE. As sane as you and I? Perhaps not, but sane enough.

Ten to two. Only two who were not in total agreement. That's pretty fair interrater reliability. Better than is obtained on most scales of human behavior. But what were they rating? Not craziness. You can bet on that one.

I'm proud of you. Of course you knew the Critchley story. I used it in *Sins of Omission*. I even gave him credit. I try to make my one milieu act for two. Or at least to replace the missing one. It doesn't really work, but it is the best I have.

You, too, must have that same possibility. Believe it or not, all those very bright guys who competed to get into medical school are still bright. I know that they hide that fact very well but their intelligence is still there below the surface if you can only scratch deep enough. If they will let you get down to it. Most won't. Some will. Especially the really intelligent ones. The Critchleys of the world of OB and gynecology.

Often the brightest do have the most interesting stories to tell. Or they tell them better. In either case, just listen and gather them in. They make your job easier. But there are stories to be gathered from everyone. Even in the billing office. Trust me.

Roger

February 14

Dear Rob,

I don't deny that there are people who have been helped by psycho-analysis. Some of my best friends have been analyzed. A few are still being analyzed. One or two fall into both groups. Analysis past and present. Certainly some people are helped by analysis. Including some of my friends. Past and present.

So what? Some people are helped by medicine men. Indian medicine men, I mean. Shamans. Does that mean that their philosophic/religious basis is valid?

The apparent efficacy of psychoanalysis in such individual cases has nothing whatsoever to do with the supposed validity of psychoanalytic theory. It does not confirm it any more than its lack of universal effica-cy refutes it. Outcome data is, in fact, silent on the issue of validity of the theory. Any physician who ever took a course in pharmacology ought to understand that. Remember all those courses you slept through in med-ical school?

Let's consider Dilantin. One of the most widely used and effective of all the anticonvulsants. No one doubts the efficacy of Dilantin. Which used to be called diphenylhydantoin, DPH for those who like acronyms, but is now known as phenytoin. Or PHT for short. But what's in a name?

Dilantin was introduced in 1938 by Putnam and Merritt. Merritt was one of America's leading neurologists. A great name in the field. DPH, later to become PHT, was the first truly new anticonvulsant to be introduced since phenobarbital, and that had taken place in 1912. It was, to understate the obvious, a major addition to our armamentarium. One of the great break-throughs, worthy of a Nobel Prize. Or at least consideration for one.

How did Dilantin work? How did it stop seizures? Putnam and Merritt knew the answer. Dilantin worked by blocking the tonic component of the seizure. By changing the nature of the abnormal electrical discharge. That's what the discoverers said. Merritt and Putnam. That's what I learned in medical school. So did you.

But they were wrong. Real wrong. Other drugs that did that were use-less in treating epilepsy.

How does it work?

Theories have come and gone. For a while, Dilantin worked because it increased the activity of the sodium pump. Then it increased cerebel-lar inhibition. Now it seems to inhibit SHFRE For the unitiated, that's sustained high frequency rapid firing. Or perhaps it decreases calcium mediated release of neurotransmitters. On the other hand, PHT also. . . . But why go on?

Clinically, it makes no difference. That's the wonderful thing about drugs—they don't have to understand their mechanism of action to have an effect. They just do whatever it is that they do without any regard for the state of knowledge of the treating physician.

That's what the whole implant story is all about. Does the process work? Not, do the adrenal cells survive? Not, do they make dopamine? Not, do the implants work by causing an inflammatory response? Those are all interesting questions, interesting issues. Good science. But not what matters.

Are Garcia's patients better? Healthier? Closer to normal? Less disabled? Less parkinsonian? Are ours? Will they stay that way? Do implants work? For how long? Not as a theoretical issue, but as a practical one.

The same is true of Eldepryl. Not, how does it slow the progression of Parkinson's disease? But does it? We believe that it does. That's what our study demonstrated. Landau didn't buy our conclusion. We, it seems, have been judged, without benefit of a jury. That's worse than being flummoxed. Far worse. "We" is the PSG, you remember the PSG, the Parkinson Study Group. Well, the PSG just had a meeting in Tampa. No, we did not meet in a bucket shop, despite Landau's comment and, no, we did not design any new pyramid schemes or Panzi schemes. Or any other kind of swindle. It was one of our regularly scheduled meetings. Our agenda was supposed to center around our next research project, but all we talked about was Landau and his attack on us all. Everyone was angry. And rightly so. But the anger should be directed at *Neurology* and its editor. Landau has a right to his opinion. It's *Neurology* that published it. They let him say we ran pyramid schemes in a bucket shop. And they published it without the usual peer review. Every other article, it seems, is refereed, judged by peers. Not this one.

So two days were spent putting together our answer and my opening line was rebuffed. So was my title. I wanted to call it "All Authors Are Created Equal." And open with the line "But William Landau is more equal than others." Or vice versa. I, too, have studied my Orwell.

They rejected my proposal. Why? Maybe they haven't read Orwell. We sent in our response. So tell your mother not to cancel her subscription to *Neurology*. Not yet, at least.

Roger

February 18

Dear Rob,

I'm now zero for five. Not a good sign. Even my first neurologic paper only went through four submissions. I now have five strikes. That's what I like about this game. You get more than three strikes. All three publishers to whom my agent submitted *The Blind Observer* as part of his brilliantly designed simultaneous multiple submissions, that's the term in the trade, have rejected it. All three. That makes it five for five. Or, more correctly, I am now nothing for five, a hitless wonder. I know the Hitless Wonders won in the end. That was the nickname of the '06 White Sox, who despite their anemic batting averages beat the Cubs in the '06 World Series.

But, as my agent reminded me, there's always another publisher out there. And he has a master plan. Let us hope that this plan is more successful than his simultaneous multiple submissions plan turned out to be. He wants us to hold an auction. I'm supposed to make nineteen fresh copies of the book and he'll submit them to nineteen other publishers simultaneously. One per publisher. The publishers will be told that they are each one of an unspecified number of publishers who have been chosen (honored) to read the manuscript and they will be given a specific date on which to make their competitive offer, to bid for my book. Just like a real auction. Not Christie's. Not Sotheby's. But nonetheless an auction. So now I have to make all those copies. Or rather my secretary has to. I do have a great day job.

I feel like a prize pig. Let's hope I sell as well. I hope I do not suffer the same fate as Van Gogh's *Tulips*. You must remember all the hoopla. It was auctioned by Sotheby's and it went for fifty three million dollars. Not bad for one modest sized canvas that is certainly not his outstanding masterpiece. Fifty three million dollars. An all-time auction record. Like Roger Maris's sixty-one home runs. Of Joe DiMaggio's fifty-six game hitting streak—ended by some guy who just happened to be named Ken Keltner.

Except it was never sold. It was all done with mirrors. Mirrors and paper transfers. The winning bidder was some Australian billionaire. Make that ex-billionaire. He won the auction but . . . and it's a big BUT. He was not bidding with real money. Sotheby's lent him the money interest-free. A paper transfer. No cash involved. Then he went belly-up and there was Sotheby's left with Van Gogh's *Tulips*, which had set the record for highest price ever. Or was it the lowest?

So hopefully I'll do better than good ol' Vincent. I'd really like to get up to .500. I wonder what my agent's average is? I have no idea. I didn't know enough to ask when I was interviewing agents. I assumed they all hit equally well. Like scientific investigators. What an assumption. As if all managers were the same. I'd love to find out. Someday.

Do I need a new agent? If I had to do it over, would I pick the same agent? I have no idea. Would I write the same books? Sell them to the same publishers? Liz Taylor said it best. She was once asked if she had to do it over, would she do the same things? Yes, but with different people.

Roger

February 24

Randall Jackson
Miskus, Smalley and Cavaretta, P.C.
Chicago, IL 60051

Dear Randy:

I was most interested in Marvelous Marty's list of his proposed expert witnesses. One of his experts is especially intriguing. Herb Klaff is probably the best known and best respected baseball writer in Chicago. He's edited several books on baseball-related literature. Not sports columns. Real literature that included baseball. Not just the name of some ballplayer, but baseball with a capital B. The opening scene of *The Chosen*. That sort of thing. Klaff probably knows more about the White Sox than any other living male. Or female for that matter. And all other Chicago sports teams. The Cubs. The Bears. The Bulls. The Blackhawks. Even the old Chicago Cardinals. Before they moved to St. Louis, from which they then moved to Phoenix, they were the Chicago Cardinals and they played their home games in Comiskey Park.

Ask Herb Klaff about Marshall Goldberg. That is the perfect question for the ideal expert witness.

Why?

We must have him, as an editor, state whether or not Marty's rights are any greater than Marshall's.

They aren't. They can't be. Herb Klaff will have to agree.

If Marty owns the name Martin Bloom, then Marshall Goldberg must own his name. If Marshall does not, how can Marty? He can't. Klaff will have to say that Marshall has the same rights. In legal terms that would have to mean that if I'd used Marshall's name, he could be suing me. That's the point I made in my deposition.

Why?

Because I have a sworn affidavit from Marshall Goldberg that I can use his name.

So what?

I'll tell you. It's not from Marshall Goldberg, halfback, Chicago Cardinals and all-American, University of Pittsburgh. Of Christman, Trippi Harder, and Goldberg fame. The Dream Backfield.

It's from Marshall Goldberg, pediatrician, Los Angeles, California. He was my next-door neighbor in the army in 1965. We were both stationed at the same army hospital, DeWitt Army Hospital, on Fort Belvoir, just outside of Washington, D.C.

I like it.

Please list as our experts the twelve baseball memorabilia dealers whose cards I am enclosing. And after we take Klaff's deposition, add one more. Marshall Goldberg. But don't tell them which Marshall Goldberg.

Roger

cc: Rob

February 26

Dear Rob,

There is no way that I can give you advice that would have any validity at all. You will have to make this choice all by yourself. The core issue is whether anyone can give valid advice as to which of the country's many writers' workshops would be best for you. I know I can't; but can anyone? After all, few, if any, of those who may so blithely answer your question for you have actually attended more than one workshop, so how could they judge them? Compare them? I have no idea.

It is the same issue you have faced before, more than once: which internship should you take? Which residency?

Medical students ask me these questions with a nauseating frequency. They think that I should be in a position to help them out of their quandary. I am, after all, the director of the neurology residency here. I empathize with their quandary. It is an important decision. It only affects, as I remind them, the rest of their lives. But what can I tell them? I only personally took segments of two residencies, neither of which I would recommend to anyone. So I really can't judge other programs. What do I really know about them? I know some of the directors and a few scattered faculty members of the larger programs. I've met a few selected graduates. Not much more. Not enough to give sound advice. But I'm supposed to be able to help them.

So I give them the following advice. Advice that few others give. Advice. Not data. Not an answer to their question, but a way of reaching an answer on their own. They should make sure that neurology is the field they want to pursue. Do they really want to take a neurology residency? Do they really want to be a neurologist?

So, Rob, do *you* really want to be a writer? The same question. A would-be neurologist must take a neurology residency, but must a would-be writer take a writer's workshop? Of course not. I never took a single course in "creative writing." Not ever. I know, it probably shows. In all the cracks.

Will a workshop make you a better writer? Or merely a different writer? If that. So should you take one? Yes. Why? To test your commitment. To learn about yourself as a writer. To begin to learn self-discipline.

So which one? I'll tell you what I tell the medical students. The one that hinders you the least. The one that wastes the least amount of your time, the one that places the fewest obstacles in your way.

How do you find that out? Ask. Who? Somebody who has taken each workshop. The workshops will give you the names. Call those people and ask them these questions. Does the workshop waste any of my time? Is it an extension of the ego of the instructor? The same questions you'd now ask about a residency. I'm willing to bet no one else ever has. It'll make them think seriously before they answer.

The workshop is like a residency. It will, if you're the right person doing the right thing, at anywhere but the wrong place, give you a chance to develop into yourself. That's all you can expect. Make sure it won't prevent that.

My good friend Bill Brashler took the workshop at Iowa. I'm sure he'll be happy to tell you all about it. I'd love to hear what he tells you. I've never asked him any questions. It was not an issue I wanted to explore.

But be warned: he's a real writer. He writes for a living. Writing for him is not a game. He knows about things like style. And tone. And voice. And the differences. His first book, *The Bingo Long Travelling Black All Stars*, was made into a movie. It's going to be reprinted this year. It's about a group of professional black baseball players in the '30s. It was published in 1973, long before black baseball was in, before blacks got into the Hall of Fame based on what they did in the black leagues. It required a lot of research on his part.

All part of the game.

Good luck,

Roger

And, yes, I knew that Shelley's *Frankenstein* was an epistolary novel. I didn't know that the right word was epistolary. I thought it was epistilatory. The editor caught it, sort of. So was *Werther*.

On second thought, you may be on the right track. Sylvia Plath, it is said, took a creative writing class after she was an accomplished, published author. When the instructor asked her why she was taking the course, she replied that she was lonesome and wanted someone to talk to.

Was that her depression? Or the loneliness of a solitary writer? A damn good question, that. And it sure as hell wasn't all her husband's fault.

Roger

March

Dostoevski's aura was a very religious feeling of immense joy and eternal harmony. So intense that he could bear it only for a few seconds, but so important that he would have sacrificed ten years of his life rather than give it up.

Dostoevski was sure that Muhammad, who had seizures, had the same experience, that Muhammad's experience in paradise had been an attack of epilepsy. Unfortunately, our patient is more prosaic. But just think: if Dostoevski was right and Muhammad's trip to paradise was a seizure, the right doctor with a little bit of phenobarbital could have changed the course of history.

Harold L. Klawans
Sins of Commission

March 1

Dear Rob,

We took Donovan's deposition today. Not the old White Sox left-handed pitcher. That Donovan won seventy-three games for us. That's almost one win for each inning Marty Bloom ever pitched. We traded him to Washington. Then he was shipped to Cleveland. He won twenty games for the Indians in '62. He was a pretty good pitcher. And a fairly good hitter. He hit fifteen home runs in his career. Did Marty ever even get a hit? He sure as heck never hit a home run. And we never used him as a pinch hitter.

No matter; it was the other Donovan. The senior editor for Sharp Books. Both are real Donovans. There can be more than one Donovan in the same reality.

The first issue was who called whom. Did I call him? Or did he call me? His lawyer felt this was a key issue. So did mine. That meant that both of the lawyers I'm paying agreed on something other than to whom to send their respective bills. Donovan said I had called him.

How had I known he was still working for Sharp Books?

He had no idea. He, by the way, still works for Sharp. That hardly makes him an unbiased witness. I know; I'm not exactly a disinterested observer, but I am above reproach. This is my book.

How had I known he was editing my book?

Again, he had no idea. But, as best as he could remember, I had called him. He wasn't certain why I had called him and readily admitted that I had not called him previously.

Had I had any correspondence with him about the book? Any contact at all? Not that he could remember.

So why had I called him?

By the way, I didn't ask any of these questions. Randy Jackson did. So I became a third person impersonal with a title, either Doctor or Professor Kramer. All formal and polite.

Why had Professor Kramer telephoned him? To tell him about the names. That, he guessed, was the real motive behind the call.

Had he read the book? Yes.

Carefully? Yes.

As an editor? Yes.

Did he have any idea, before the phone call, that I had used names that also belonged to baseball players? No. Not even an inkling.

Randy saw his chance and moved in. "You edited this book?" he asked.

"Yes," Donovan agreed.

"So you read each and every line very carefully?"

Another yes.

Had he read my chapter "Dead Arm Dick?" He had.

The paragraphs about the use of names of baseball players? Where I wrote about Allison Kozar? Where I explained that Al Kozar had been reborn as a woman? Yes.

Had he read the next chapter? He had.

What was the name of the medical student in that chapter?

He didn't remember.

My lawyer read him the appropriate paragraph. The name, of course, was Allison Kozar. Did that refresh his memory?

It did.

As an editor, didn't that remind him of what I'd written just ten pages earlier about Allison Kozar being a variation of the name of Al Kozar?

He wasn't sure.

I told you, you can't depend on editors. Even Hemingway couldn't. Hemingway, by the way, supposedly owed much of his style to his experience as a journalist. In *The Sun Also Rises*, his first great novel, he mentioned Frankie Frisch, one of baseball's outstanding second basemen, who was later elected to the Baseball Hall of Fame. Frisch, known as the Fordham Flash, was a graduate of Fordham. He played for the New York Giants. They later traded him to the St. Louis Cardinals for Rogers Hornsby, another future Hall of Fame second baseman, a better hitter but not as good a fielder. The point. In *The Sun Also Rises*, he misspelled Frisch's name. So much for his experience as a journalist. And so much for the contribution of his editor.

Roger

March 6

Dear Rob,

It came like a bolt out of the blue. Or an unexpected home run from some anemic batter. That was a nice mixed metaphor with a touch of the medical thrown in. And it started out so innocently, like most rallies and all too many serious diseases. We have someone new working in our office. This is a big department. Eighteen neurologists and a support staff at least twice that big. So new employees are hired with a surprising frequency. And I get introduced to each of them, paying very little attention to most of these *pro forma* invitations. Her name, I was told, was Cassie. Was that her real name or just what she was called, I wondered. It was a warm, sunny afternoon, quite sunny and warm for late February here in Chicago. It was one of those days that reeked of Spring training, a day that, to me, was redolent of the cracks of bats hitting balls. The kind of day that dreams are made of. If Hammett can steal from the Bard, I can too.

Cassie, I said to myself, hoping to remember the name. Or Cassy? Or did she spell it with a K? She was a new billing clerk. She was tall, young, willowy, blond. Taller than anyone else in the billing office, she was about my height. Five foot ten. She was also younger than any of our other billing clerks. Twenty at the outside, and more willowy and a lot blonder. I resisted the temptation to look down at her legs. My mind was filled with questions. How long would she last? What kind of a job was being a billing clerk in a doctor's office for a tall, young, willowy blond named . . . Cassie? Or Kassy?

Cassie, I decided. But how to remember her name? As always, by association. Cass Michaels. He'd been the White Sox second baseman when I'd first become a Sox fan. Cass Michaels had not been his real name. He had been christened Casimir Eugene Kwietniewski. And in 1949 he'd hit .308. Cassie as in Cass Michaels. And Cassandra. A tall, willowy, blond, young seer. Had Cassandra ever been that young? She had been ageless. Who knew her age? Age was not one of her determining characteristics.

She walked off to the billing office and I went back to seeing patients. And gave neither her nor her name any further thought. I didn't even hear her name again for several days and when I finally did, it had been magically transformed. I heard it over our overhead loudspeaker system, almost like being paged at a ball park. "Cassandra. . . ." I was right. Her name was Cassandra. One for the good guys. The face that launched a thousand ships. Wrong face. Right war.

"Cassandra Waitkus, ..."

Waitkus. WAITKUS! A name that launched a thousand memories. One memory. One indelible memory. One of baseball's most enduring memories. Eddie Waitkus. First baseman. Chicago Cubs and Philadelphia Phillies. *The Natural*. Not really, but Malamud's prototype for one enduring scene, a single indelible image. The model on whom the natural was based. A baseball player shot in a hotel room by a female fan. That really happened. Right here in Chicago. In the old Edgewater Beach Hotel. And it happened to Eddie Waitkus. It took place in '49, when he was playing for the Phillies. The Cubs had traded him to Philadelphia. He was one of the Whiz Kids. And the Phillies were in town to play the Cubs. The team was staying at the Edgewater Beach Hotel. A young woman came up to his room.

Her name? I remembered—Ruth something or other. Ruth Steinhagen, I think.

Her age? Not as clear. Probably around twenty. Or younger. Ruth Steinhagen shot Eddie Waitkus in a hotel room. A tender spot. One shot in the chest. He missed the rest of the season. That might have cost the Phillies the pennant. They won in '50 with Waitkus playing first base.

Ruth Steinhagen was from Chicago. Single. A secretary, I think. A fan. And she was the heavy in the story. She shot Eddie Waitkus. He was the ballplayer. He was the hero. The good guy. Clean-cut. Pure. Chaste. She was the bad guy. To shoot a player, she had to be deranged. To say the least. She was arrested. He came to her hotel room and she shot him.

A trial? Had there been a trial? I seemed to remember something about her being in a mental institution of some sort. Declared crazy. End of case.

Today, of course, it might all turn out so differently. Or at least it would all be perceived so differently. Her defense would be obvious. She'd plead self-defense! She was just a poor, trusting, naive girl. Eddie had seemed so nice. So clean-cut. All she had wanted was his autograph. And then. . . . My God, she hadn't invited him there for that. She was a nice girl. She tried to resist. What choice did she have? He was all over her. Like Mike Tyson. Only faster. He'd be the one who would be arrested. With no chance to cop an insanity plea.

I went into the billing office. There she was.

"Cassandra Waitkus," I said.

"Yes?"

"Are you related to Eddie Waitkus?" I asked. "*The* Eddie Waitkus," I added superfluously.

"Yes," she nodded, "he was my grandfather's first cousin."

Was. "Is he dead?"

"Yes."

"I remember him," I said.

"The Natural," she smiled.

"The Natural." I said. "Roy Hobbs. Good brought down by evil. Good that later had to try to redeem itself. Good. Purity. . . . You know," I went on. "I was brought up to believe that there was a certain innocence to the original story. That Eddie was an innocent victim. That he was pure. I hope I'm not insulting you or your family. I don't know what your family believes; but I no longer believe that it was all quite that innocent."

She looked at me, smiled as one would at a child who had just discovered a fact that every adult already knew. "Neither do we," she said. "Neither do we."

There are stories, even in the billing office, Rob. Just like I told you. The process consists of listening to the stories and figuring out which ones are worth telling. And then figuring out how to best tell these stories. And, of course, to do the footwork, the research. I haven't done that. This is just what I remembered. Nothing more. Will I do more? Probably not. I'm not writing about Eddie Waitkus. Besides, he can't sue me; he's dead.

Why couldn't that have happened to Martin Bloom? And not just in my book?

Roger

March 7

Dear Rob,

My review came out today, for those of us who subscribe to the *New York Times Book Review*. The rest of the readership will see it on Sunday. Or get it on Sunday and get around to reading it sometime after Sunday, hopefully before the next one arrives. It's pretty much like the letter to you, although I added a bit to make the traditional view of handedness more apparent to the non-medical reader. After all, Rob, you may be a gynecologist, but you did study neurology once. Most readers never did. So I explained the traditional neurologic wisdom, which maintains that left-handedness is usually a hereditary nuisance, not a medical condition. Most readers are probably unaware that handedness, especially left-handedness, is basically a neurologic issue. One of the first questions a neurologist asks any patient is about his or her handedness. If the patient is right-handed, it ends there. If he or she is left-handed, then two possibilities are entertained: left-handedness on a hereditary basis versus left-handedness because of damage to the left hemisphere of the brain. After all, it is the brain, not the limb, that determines handedness, and the left hemisphere directs the right hand and vice versa. Speech is usually a function of the left or dominant hemisphere and in most individuals that left hemisphere becomes dominant for handedness. Anatomically, this is not surprising. The motor areas directing the hand are in close juxtaposition to the speech areas. Physiologically, it is also not surprising. We are not just handed for the way we throw a baseball or hammer a nail, but also for handwriting and those hand gestures associated with speech. Such gestures long antedate writing. Man is also right-handed for signing. The left hemisphere is the home base of sign language.

So the neurologist follows up the issue. Is anyone else in your family left-handed? "No." That response raises the specter of "pathologic" left-handedness, left-handedness because of injury (pathologic change) in the left hemisphere that has prevented it from doing its usual job. It is a "no" that is filled with neurologic meaning.

But most patients say "yes." And there it ends. Hereditary left-handedness, we think to ourselves. No brain damage. Nothing pathologic. Merely a social, educational, and occupational nuisance. A lifetime of scissors that don't fit right (no pun intended), electrical appliances with switches in the wrong places, cars with gear shifts on the wrong side, and a world without left-handed catchers' mitts. A distinctly underrated form of discrimination. To say nothing of the problem it causes in learning to write.

The editor came up with a great title. "Don't Wait for Lefty—He's Dead." Does anyone still read *Waiting for Lefty*? When was it last produced?

I learned another thing. The *New York Times* only refers to physicians as doctors. Coren is a Ph.D. He has a doctorate degree. I referred to him as Dr. Coren. They changed it to Mr. Coren. I found that rather peculiar. But then so is the reverse policy that refers to Castro as Dr. Castro because he has, it is said, a doctorate degree in law.

Roger

March 13

Dear Rob,

We've completed nine implants now. They've all been operated on and have all been discharged from the hospital. We'll probably do a few more. Perhaps an even dozen. Not the result of some fancy power analysis. A dozen will be enough for us. Not for the patients, but enough for us. We will have the answers we need. Or at least some of them. That may say it all. You don't decide to stop performing miracles. I never quit giving levodopa.

No one has been cured. The patients are all a bit better but they have not been resurrected. There is still a need for a new Lourdes. Our job now is to study these patients and try to figure out why they have improved. We still don't know why the implants work at all. As far as we can tell, the cells probably don't survive and even if they do they don't make enough dopamine to cause a significant degree of improvement. But the patients do improve. Now we need to know why. Back to the lab. And we also don't know how long the improvement will last. That is a clinical question. Only time will give us the answer.

Many scientists have been critical of us. They have not said that we've been operating in a bucket shop. Or have been carrying out Panzi schemes. But critical nonetheless. Mostly it's been the basic scientists. The ones who have been studying implants in their labs. Many of them believe that we acted prematurely. That we had jumped the gun. More preliminary work should have been done on animals. Perhaps we have moved too quickly, but what choice did we have? Garcia had thrown down a challenge. A public gauntlet, if ever there was one. It had to be pursued. We had no other choice. Besides, our patients did all right. The implants are working to some degree and that success has been intoxicating.

I was in Sweden for three days. I presented our results. The Swedes are the ones who started the whole implant business. They had never believed Garcia's results. To them the *NEJM* is just another American journal in a world filled with far too many such journals. So I presented our results to the pioneers in brain implants. Was I bringing coals to Newcastle? Or atomic energy? They were impressed. It had not just been coals. There was something to this implant business after all.

I got back yesterday, and today a physician from Pennsylvania was flown in to see us. He has Parkinson's disease. He'd been treating himself for years. He'd seen the article in the *New England Journal of Medicine*. To him, it was not just another journal and not just another research report. He finished work that day and walked out of his office and flew off to Mexico City to see Garcia, and within days he had undergone the surgery and he has been confused ever since. He's now totally disabled. Unable to take care of himself, much less practice medicine. Because of his confusion, not his Parkinson's. That had never been bad enough to interfere with his practice. He'd obviously had a severe brain injury from surgery. Albright revisited. You remember Albright. If not, see my letter of whatever date it was. I'm keeping all my copies. Are you? But I do not have an index.

He'd had a major surgical complication. Could we help him? After all, his surgery had been successful. Who'd said that? Garcia himself, we were told.

I haven't heard from Fred Gould in a while. Nothing unusual about that. Last I heard, he was going to see Garcia. Off to Mecca. How's that for mixing metaphors?

David came by yesterday and gave me another book to read, a collection of letters by Edward Dahlberg. My letters to you reminded him of Dahlberg's letters. The same sort of quirkiness of style and opinion. So I began to read them. The best part was the *errata* card. First it informed me that the writer Marston mentioned on page sixty-nine was not Bourke Marston, who had been cited in the footnote, but the Elizabethan author John Marston. Having never heard of either, I was unmoved by this error on the part of the editor. Not so the next one. There I learned that *Legends of the Jews*, which the editor had identified as written by Allen Ginsberg had been written not by the author of *Howl*, but by the noted Jewish scholar Louis Ginzberg.

How's that for a mistake by an editor? Sort of like confusing Grover Cleveland with Glover Cleveland Alexander. The latter was the Hall of Fame pitcher. The former needs no identification. Or vice versa. And you thought that a good editor would solve all your problems.

Clarence Darrow once called Louis Ginzberg. Not to discuss *Howl*, you can bet on that. Why? To ask him about Cain's wife. Recall the scene in *Inherit the Wind*. Clarence Darrow is questioning William Jennings Bryan. He had called Ginzberg about that question. Cain's wife. Where did she come from? Was there some other creation going on next-door? The only inhabitants in Eden were Adam, Eve, and Cain. Abel was dead. It was the Sabbath, so Ginzberg wouldn't talk on the phone. His wife did. And he agreed to send Darrow the appropriate pages from *Legends of the Jews*.

Yes, David knows that I'm compiling a collection of letters. He's already read the first couple of months. That means he knows that I haven't read any of his short stories and have been waiting for him to ask me to read them. I'm still waiting. He has made some suggestions, some of which I will probably heed. Which ones, I'll never tell.

Dahlberg wrote to a group of interesting people: Theodore Dreiser, Robert M. Hutchins, William Carlos Williams, Herbert Read, Lewis Mumford. . . . The list goes on. I write to you. His letters got published. I also write to Medicare, insurance companies, suppliers of wheelchairs, visiting nursing services, the Illinois Department of Public Aid. Not exactly Theodore Dreiser. Not even Upton Sinclair.

I got a letter today from a pediatric neurologist from Montreal named Michael Schevell. He had read my article about Birkmayer and also a clinical tale of mine about a German neurologist named Hallervorden. Hallervorden did neuropathologic studies on victims killed in the Nazi "euthanasia" program. When confronted as to his use of such material, he remarked, "There was wonderful material among those brains, beautiful mental defectives, malformations and early infantile diseases. I accepted those brains of course. Where they came from and how they came to me was really none of my business." NONE OF MY BUSINESS. Now there's a line for you. You could build an entire novel on that as a last line. The way Malamud did with *The Natural*. Transforming "Say it ain't so, Joe" into "Say it ain't so, Roy."

Schevell has published a scholarly paper on Hallervorden. He also sent me his newest paper. It's about another German neurologist named Schaltenbrand. Schaltenbrand injected spinal fluid from patients with multiple sclerosis into various individuals who were forced to participate. The purpose was to see if MS was caused by a virus. The experiments were not done in some death camp, but at the University of Würzburg.

And in 1955 he was elected an Honorary Member of the American Neurological Association. I may resign. Or merely be sick.

Roger

March 13

Austin Flint, M.D., President
American Neurological Association

Dear Sir:

Enclosed please find a paper by Michael Schevell detailing the illegal, immoral, unethical, and undoubtedly criminal activities of one Georges Schaltenbrand.

I demand that his Honorary Membership be revoked immediately and his name be stricken from our official records.

> *Roger Kramer*
>
> *Fellow*
> *American Neurological Association*

cc: Rob

P.S. Rob. He's been dead for twenty years. At least the Inquisition had nothing on me. I won't demand an auto da fé.

March 14

Dear Rob,

I woke up with a chill last night. I'd just remembered Schaltenbrand's major post-war accomplishment. It was an atlas of the brain done on normal, perfectly preserved, totally undistorted human brains. Most of the work was done in Chicago by a neuropathologist named Percival Bailey. The brains had been brought here from Germany. Flown in. Right after the war.

Percival Bailey was President of the ANA when Schaltenbrand was given his Honorary Membership and defended Schaltenbrand from all charges when his work was attacked in an American journal.

Now where do you think Schaltenbrand got those brains? Those normal brains? Those normal human brains? Those totally undistorted, normal human brains? Those perfectly preserved, totally undistorted, normal human brains? Any good guesses?

They had to have been removed almost instantaneously after death. Think about that. No, don't. You may wake up with chills.

What difference does posthumously stripping him of an honor make to anyone? We are not the Inquisition. We have no absolute authority.

Roger

March 16

Dear Rob,

My God, you would have thought that I had written the damn book, not merely a rather brief review of it. All I did was put together some seven hundred and fifty words, but ever since that review appeared on Sunday I have been inundated by phone calls and letters, most from left-handers proclaiming that their mere existence (i.e., being alive) proves that I am wrong. Could I apply that logic to *Bloom vs. Me et al.*? Does not his mere existence prove that I was not writing about him?

But I didn't write the book. I didn't do the research. And a few survivors mean nothing. I know it means a lot to each of the survivors, but not the statistician.

The best letter came from William Glazer of Yale. He's an Associate Professor of Psychiatry there and is in charge of their Tardive Dyskinesia Clinic. Tardive dyskinesia is a side effect of antipsychotic drugs like Thorazine and Haldol. After patients take these for years, some of them develop tardive dyskinesia. Tardive dyskinesia is a neurologic disorder. It consists of abnormal movements. That's what "dyskinesia" means: abnormal movement. And "tardive" means late. Abnormal movements that come on late in the use or after prolonged use of these antipsychotic drugs. It's one of the disorders I've been studying for years. It's one of the major problems in psychiatry today. These drugs revolutionized the treatment of schizophrenia. Before them, the average length of stay in an institution for an acute schizophrenic attack was two years. Look at Nijinsky. He had his psychotic break in the late teens and was institutionalized for decades. Now it's twenty-one days or less.

But some patients get these movements, and in some of them the movements are severe, contorting, disabling. A dilemma.

Dr. Glazer had read my review. That prompted him to write to me about a research finding of theirs. Perhaps I could explain it. They have been following an outpatient group of some four hundred patients since 1985 and have identified over eighty patients in that group with tardive dyskinesia. Their five-year risk of tardive dyskinesia is thirty-two percent and their estimated twenty-five year risk is sixty-eight percent. They decided to check their patients to see if handedness was a risk factor. Their hypothesis was that left-handed people, unfortunate in every other way, would have a higher rate of tardive dyskinesia. If left-handedness represents some sort of brain injury, this would not be unexpected. To their surprise, they found that left-handers were *protected* from developing tardive dyskinesia. In their study left-handers had only one-third the risk that right-handers did. It was better to be left-handed. An unexpected result.

Did I have any explanation? They didn't. I'm supposed to be the expert. I discovered the first animal model of tardive dyskinesia and that was twenty years ago. Have I learned anything in twenty years? I hope so.

Roger

March 19—London

Dear Rob,

That's right, London. But not for long. A couple of days. Two days and one night in between and then a short stop in Amsterdam and then home. Believe me, Rob, being a jet setter sounds far more glamorous than it is. I had to go to London for a project related to Parkinson's disease. The old problem of rating scales. Any investigator who studies Parkinson's disease must use scales to measure the symptoms such as tremor, slowness of movement, what have you. Most of us use one particular scale, called the UPDRS. That's short for the Unified Parkinson's Disease Rating Scale. Another acronym. We in medicine produce as many as the New Deal ever did. In PD we use the UPDRS. Not Garcia, of course, but most of the rest of us. It was put together by a team of neurologists led by Stan Fahn from Columbia. The scale rates each symptom from 0 to 4. And describes what 1, 2, 3, and 4 mean. Zero is always normal. And 4+ is always maximal. The worst possible tremor. The greatest rigidity. But those descriptions are written descriptions. Words. Words that can be interpreted differently by different readers. That's fine for literature, but not for experimental medicine. What does a 2+ tremor really look like? Or 3+ foot taps?

Do the experts agree? Do I see the same 2+ tremor that Stan does? Or is my 2+ sometimes a 3+ to him? Or the other way around? Do I use the criteria the same way he does? Or David Marsden, the acknowledged European expert on PD? Do the others investigators know exactly what 2+ means to the three of us? A number of good questions. The solution? Put together hundreds of brief videotaped excerpts of patients, show them to the experts and have them rate the tapes, then put together a single video made up of those snippets on which we all independently agreed. So that's what we did in London. Arnold Chiari put together hundreds of brief segments and Stan, David, and I rated them. For eight hours. It was exhausting. And now Arnold has the job of going over the results. Let's hope we agreed often enough so that we don't have to do it again.

Once we were finished, I bid them all farewell and went to dinner with Dannie and Joan Abse. Dannie is one of the leading British poets. He's Welsh. He's also a physician—a chest specialist. A physician-writer. One of the very best. He is president of the Poetry Society. He just retired, from the practice of medicine, not from writing.

Do writers ever retire? Composers do stop composing. Intentionally. At the height of their careers. Rossini. Sibelius. Do writers? Or is that always called "writer's block?" You don't think of novelists retiring. Did Hemingway retire? Do playwrights? Or are they just working on plays in progress? Sort of like Boito. He burst on the operatic world with a masterpiece, *Mefistofele*, and spent the rest of his life writing his second opera, *Nerone*. It was not worth that much effort. He did write a couple of librettos along the way. Great ones. Otello. Falstaff. He took from the best better than anyone else did. But we're discussing his operas here, not Verdi's.

Dannie no longer practices medicine. As a result, he now has more time to write. He has retired into writing, so to speak. A fantasy come true.

At dinner, we were joined by William and Patricia Oxley. William is a poet. Don't feel bad, Rob. I, too, had never heard of him. He's even written an epic poem, *A Map of Time*. A published epic. I didn't know anyone since Kazantzakis had written an epic, much less gotten one published. And certainly I had never met anyone who wrote an epic. Homer, Virgil, Anonymous, and William Oxley. Is *Paterson* an epic? William Carlos Williams' long poem. Or is it just a very long poem? There is a difference.

Patricia edits a literary magazine, *Acumen*. I love the name. Clinical acumen is what we strive for in our lives as physicians. That's where it's at. Clinical acumen. To her as an editor, critical acumen is the key. Mature, careful, impersonal judgment. Judgment based on knowledge and experience. I never think of acumen in that non-clinical sense. Acumen is not a medical word per se. No more than words like pernicious or miliary.

"How did you start a journal?" I asked.

"We owe it all to Matthew Arnold," William informed me.

It seems that in his youth, William had collected a few letters or other documents signed by poets like Matthew Arnold and Alexander Pope. They'd been cheap then. A few shillings apiece. That's why he bought them. A letter by Matthew Arnold for next to nothing, the cost of fish and chips. And no grease. That was in the days before the craze for collecting autographs of great writers. Times have changed. People collect everything now. I know. I mentioned that my daughter collects Fiesta ware. None of them had any idea what that was. I tried to explain. William was certain that I wouldn't believe how valuable such autographs had become.

I would. He wouldn't believe what old baseball cards are worth today. Mickey Mantle's rookie card. And I once owned it. I had the complete set of 1951. And 1950. And 1952. And . . . a rookie Mickey Mantle. Now there is a real collector's item. Hell, no Matthew Arnold ever cost that much. Or ever would.

And think of that famous Honus Wagner cigarette card! The most valuable of all baseball cards. The *Tulips* of baseball cards. No one has ever seen a signed one. A signed *Iliad* would cost less.

Eight years ago William sold his entire collection of by then valuable literary autographs and they had enough money to start the magazine. If he'd had more, they'd have fewer problems keeping it going. And if I still had all my baseball cards. Mickey Mantle's rookie card. Eddie Matthews. Hank Aaron. I had them all.

They produce a run of seven hundred fifty copies of each issue of *Acumen*. And they were in London to deliver them to those half dozen bookstores that carry it. Poetry, it appears, sells no better in the U.K. than it does in the U.S. Seven hundred fifty issues! One for each of Ruth's homers with a few left over.

"Do you sell them all?" I asked.

"Oh, yes," he told me. "Some issues are out of print. Gone. They've become collector's items."

"Save some. Don't sell them all. When there is enough demand, you can sell them and buy a Matthew Arnold autograph," I said. Or a Nellie Fox rookie card. Something really valuable.

Much of the conversation centered on the state of British poetry. And individual poets. I was immediately jealous. Not that I wasn't a poet. That would be like being jealous of Michael Jordan. You can't be jealous of a talent you never really aspired to, that God completely gave to someone else. I was jealous because they all know each other. They break bread together. Or pull it apart. We were in a Nepalese restaurant pulling nan apart. And discussing poetry together. Their own works. Their works in progress. The works of others. They can sit and argue about art and aesthetics and meter and what a poem really means.

I have no such environment. No such element. And never will. I am tired of rehashing patients in the hallway, getting curbstone consults on abdominal pain. I want a curbstone consult on Matthew Arnold. I'll settle for Rilke.

They talked of David Gascoyne. He's a British poet who had an acute psychotic break some forty years ago. He'd known Dannie back then. They were young poets in a circle of young poets. Jealousy again.

Gascoyne had become increasingly withdrawn and paranoid. More and more paranoid. One night he turned to Dannie for help. A desperate knock on the door. Dannie had just finished medical school. He was about to start his day job as a doctor. But what could he do? He was not a psychiatrist.

David Gascoyne was institutionalized shortly after that. In some twentieth century Bedlam. And stayed there. Withdrawn. Catatonic. Mute. Not just a short admission. It lasted almost forty years. That was before Thorazine. Nijinsky revisited. Then a woman came by the chronic psychiatric hospital where he was institutionalized to read poems to the patients. She introduced a poem by David Gascoyne.

"I be he," a voice said.

She read the poem. And the next week, another. And David Gascoyne talked to her.

In a few months, the poet was discharged to her care. They've been married for the last six to eight years.

"Does he write poetry?" I asked.

"He does translations," I was told.

It was a strange story. Something did not ring true. He could not have really been schizophrenic. Schizophrenics did not get better after forty years. Not like that. But what?

"I talked to him about his illness once," Dannie continued. "He told me that in the '40s he was sick, but he thought he'd be better in the '50s. In the '50s he knew he was sick, but he thought he'd be better in the '60s. And so it went. And in the '80s he was better."

Before I left London, I bought a copy of the latest issue of *Acumen*. There was a review of David Gascoyne's *Journals*. His psychosis had not just happened. It had been drug-induced. He had abused amphetamines. Especially Benzedrine and Methadrine. Benzedrine was the "in" drug then. So he had had a drug-induced schizophrenic-like state. Not true schizophrenia. Not Nijinsky revisited.

I will subscribe to *Acumen*. Why? I may start a collection. I don't read much poetry. That's David Garron's thing. He is the only person I know who admits he reads poetry. It's his major passion. I don't think *Acumen* will be a great investment. Baseball cards are a better bet.

I am now on my way to Amsterdam. Or at least the first draft is being composed while I am flying from London to Amsterdam. This morning, before I left London, I was interviewed by the BBC. TV-2. They shot on camera a twenty minute long interview for their late night show. They had called me last week to tell me that they were doing a series of interviews of physician-writers. There seem to be more of us now. And in the U.K. they take us far more seriously than anyone here does. It's almost as if they believe that disease and the experience of disease means something. What a concept! They wanted to interview me and were pleased that I was coming to London and set up a studio to do the interview. The interviewer asked me why more authors are writing about disease and dying now than ever before. Not just physicians, but other writers, too.

It's a question I've thought about a lot. I think it's because the nature of death has changed and with that the experience of dying. For the first time in the history of mankind, most people will not die an acute, sudden death. That means most of us will have to come to terms with some sort of chronic disease and the death that it foreshadows. Disease is now a way of life. Not acute diseases. Not the plague. Not smallpox. We live in an era of chronic diseases. Cancer. Alzheimer's. Parkinson's. So many of the debilitating diseases. Strokes. Arthritis. And we do not experience these diseases as metaphors. Not as punishments. Not TB as the reward for a life as a courtesan. That was all right in the nineteenth century but it won't work today. Cancer in your own body is not a parallel to a cancer on the body politic. Chronic disease is now the expected reward for living. Nothing metaphoric about that. And it will happen to most of us.

It's been happening to our parents, our relatives, our friends. Sometimes even to our children. So it naturally has become the subject of literature. And we don't have that many models from other eras. Classic literature accepts death. And deaths are almost always sudden and most often it is the death of someone other than the hero. There's a lot of reaction to the deaths, but anticipation of one's own death, of contemplation of the desolation of one's own life, the loss of capacities, the onset of progressive disability, the loss of independence. Where is that dissected? Maybe the first act of *Lear*. But very few other places. And even the Bard uses deformity as a metaphor. Richard III. By the way, he had nothing to do with the death of those two boys in the tower. All Tudor propaganda. And no hump either. Evil looks as evil is. Such drivel. But even Lear is silent as to the experience of dying. So little has been written about how the world changes around the dying person, how his loved ones change, how he changes, how nothing remains the same. The desperation. The resignation. The anger. The sweetness. The frustration. How patients demand treatment. And how doctors have the same need to treat. The games we all play. The euphemisms we use.

So, of course, it has become the subject of literature. And I try to write about it. So do other physicians. We as physicians have a perspective that no non-physician has. Not better, different. We have participated in the process by choice. And unless we look away, which is what most of us do, we have the charge to observe and learn. Of course, looking away is easier. And more natural. We do not know precisely how the dying patient feels. There is no one way, no single progression, but we see the erosion of life and behavior in a naked way that no one else sees. And crises and resolutions that no novelist would ever dream up.

If we only had the skill and the time. The time you can create. The skill. Aye, there's the rub. Robert Louis Stevenson always carried two books with him wherever he went, and he went lots of places. One was to read. The other was to write in. It was not so much, he explained, that he wanted to be a writer. He wanted to learn how to write. He practiced writing to gain proficiency, to learn how to write. In the same way that other men learned how to whittle. His analogy, not mine. Nice choice, that. Whittling's invariably a self-taught skill. It always was and still is. There are no classes in whittling. No whittler's workshops. No postgraduate courses in whittling. It's a skill to be acquired through personal effort. Personal effort and self-criticism.

Roger

March 21—Flying home from Amsterdam

Dear Rob,

    I was reading an art magazine I bought in London. *Modern Painting.* There was, in it, a full page ad from the British publisher Thames and Hudson. They have just published a volume of letters by Oscar Kokoschka. O.K.'s own letters. Had any of them been written to Alma? As Alma Mahler? Or Alma Gropius? Or Alma Mahler again? Or Mrs. Werfel? Or Alma Mahler? Once more? She outlived all her husbands and always reverted to the name Mahler. And O.K. outlived her. Did he write letters to her? Literary parallels to his great paintings?

    It was easy enough to find out. Buy the book. It's not published in the U.S. Only the U.K. Order it. It's not that difficult. Nor am I that interested. David would. He would leave no source unturned to find any such letters. He would apply all of the trappings of pure scholarship. I could do that. I know all the rules as well as he does. All the mechanisms. All the tricks of the trade. But I won't be doing it. It is not that I'm tired. Or I've lost my appetite for that degree of scholarship. Not so. Not true. It's just that such an attempt would be tangential to my needs. I have seen his paintings. I know the story of his doll. That wondrous doll. These are enough for me. Sometimes data kills the story. That's what's wrong with data. It can disprove a null hypothesis. Never prove, just disprove. I'm not writing O.K.'s biography. Nor a critical study of his art. Nor Alma's autobiography. Don't confuse me with facts.

    In Amsterdam I had time to stop by the Stedlijk Museum. They had a summer show of pieces from the museum's own collection. One was a Picasso. From '42 or '43. *A Woman with a Fishhat.* A woman done in bold white and blue strokes wearing a hat featuring a fish. So this is what Picasso was doing while Max Jacob was being packed into a cattle car. On the opposite wall there was a Chiam Soutine. Soutine was a French Jew. And an artist. He died in Paris in '43. Of what? He wasn't even fifty. Not of an excess of brotherly love. On that you can bet. Nor liberté! Nor equalité! Nor fraternité!

Roger

March 25

William M. Glazer, M.D.
Director, TD Clinic
Department of Psychiatry
Yale University

Dear Dr. Glazer:

Your letter was intriguing to me and, believe it or not, I may have an explanation as to why left-handers appear to be protected from tardive dyskinesia. This explanation merely requires that we take a step back and discard one of our most tightly held prejudices; namely, that all diseases represent abnormal function. It is an assumption that is almost always valid and one we physicians believe in so strongly that we forget that it is merely an assumption on our part. It is. Give it up for a few minutes. Even before I got your letter or read Coren's book, I have toyed with the notion that tardive dyskinesia, or at least that process within the brain that results in the movements we call abnormal, is the normal response of the normal brain to the toxic insult of antipsychotic drugs. Normal. Usual. Expected. What is supposed to happen. Not abnormal. Not unusual. Not unexpected. Not what's not supposed to happen. Outrageous? I don't think so. Is lead poisoning abnormal? Of course it is. However, and this is a big however, the abnormality consists not in the altered brain function caused by the lead. That's what lead does, that's how a normal brain responds to lead. The abnormality lies in the exposure to the lead. It shouldn't be in the brain. Well, neither should antipsychotic drugs. Unless you consider schizophrenia to represent a state of abnormal Thorazine deficiency. Certainly, if you give people enough neuroleptics long enough, the majority of them actually develop tardive dyskinesia (projected to be sixty-eight percent in twenty-five years in your study). Add to this observation of yours one other observation. The patients receiving antipsychotic drugs for other reasons, who were never psychotic, can also go on to develop tardive dyskinesia, and the amount of drug that these patients received is far lower than the doses used in schizophrenics. Think about that for a minute. Schizophrenics can get TD but it takes more drugs and schizophrenics start out with an abnormal brain.

I would put this all together like this:

1. Antipsychotics, acting as a toxin on the dopaminergic receptors, produce a response in the receptor. This response is what finally causes the abnormal movements. I've been writing about that for twenty years now. Nothing new in this. The drugs act on the brain cells, causing a response.

2. This response occurs in all brains. It is a normal response. The normal response. But, like all responses, some brains respond more than others. As Orwell would have put it, some brains are more equal. Or in more scientific terms, any stimulus causes a range of responses, some greater, some lesser, but all within a normal range.

3. Tardive dyskinesia is the eventual outcome of this normal response. It's what the brain does when poisoned in this way.

4. But some brains are less equal. Even abnormally so. And that may be a good thing because those brains that are less able to generate this response would be less susceptible to tardive dyskinesia. This would include schizophrenics, all of whom have abnormal brains, and especially left-handed schizophrenics. This would be adding injury to injury, abnormality upon abnormality. In other words, the abnormality of the brain in left-handers inhibits their normal response to a toxin, and, thus, they do not develop tardive dyskinesia as often.

That was what my animal work was all about. I gave Haldol to the guinea pigs for a month and they all, *all*, ALL, one hundred percent, became changed. We'd produced a behavior that was "abnormal," like the movements in tardive dyskinesia. But was it really abnormal? How could it be? They all got it. It was normal to become abnormal in *that* particular way when given that drug. So tardive dyskinesia is *the normal response*—the expected response. A normal abnormal behavior, so to speak. That's what your research shows. If sixty-eight percent get it, that's a "normal" response. No matter how you define normal. It is the usual expected response.

While these ideas are free, I would at least hope for a "thank you" note in the research they might generate. And like any good hypothesis, this one will only be worthwhile if it generates research that tests it.

I'm glad you took the time to write me, and please give my thoughts some consideration. I don't think they are as out in left field as they initially might seem. You should be interested in knowing that you may be the only individual who wrote me in response to my review who did not proclaim his or her left-handedness in the initial letter. You may, in fact, be the only right-hander who wrote me.

The only question is whether Coren's hypothesis is true. It has yet to be directly disproven, but that doesn't mean it is true. It's merely a hypothesis. Not a truism.

Sincerely yours,

Roger Kramer, M.D.
Professor of Neurological
Sciences and Pharmacology

cc: Rob

P.S. Rob, don't show this to the secretary who is named Rob. Or do. After all, she may be educable. Or whatever you want.

March 29

Dear Rob,

So you saw our response to Landau's vicious attack in this month's issue of *Neurology*. Via your mother, I presume. And our missive seemed weak and petulant. It probably was. I'm too close to tell. The table was set against us. It was like my writing a letter to the editor of a newspaper to correct a "bad" book review. I've never done that. Except when I wrote to you. And that was a private letter between friends. Not the public outcry of a wounded pride. Whenever you do that, you appear to be a petulant adolescent, no matter how right you are. And all we got was publication as a letter to the editor, not a full article.

Enough. Life goes on. Even in the field of research. Mylan has not gone down yet. I guess most financial advisors don't have mothers who read *Neurology*. Lucky them.

The patients all still want to be on Eldepryl. They demand to be on Eldepryl. Their mothers obviously don't read *Neurology*. Or perhaps they have a need for myths. For hope. Don't we all? Let us hope our myth is true. Or at least is not proven to be untrue. Myth as hypothesis is okay, but not as disproven hypothesis. God forbid that Landau was right.

My reluctance to mention current events, my reticence, my refusal in these letters has been intentional. These letters should be timeless. Or dateless. These may be the record of this specific year in my life, but not of a specific year in the world's life. Scientific references cannot be avoided, but not many people can date these letters by such references. My colleagues can. But they will only read the book if I give them each a copy. A problem that is easily solved. Literary references are also fine. They all have a wonderful timelessness. But historical references, references to historical events are out.

But some things cannot be ignored. Here's one. It has to do with art. Fine art. There is a new form of art tours. You could be the first in your area to sign up. It's being offered by the Belgrade Tourist Bureau. It's a full day's trip from Belgrade to Vukevar. Vukevar is, or was, a lovely, picturesque, historic Croatian city on the banks of the beautiful blue Danube. It was a town that Serbian troops pounded to bits last Fall. Note I did not give the date.

There is a flier that describes the full day tour. You leave Belgrade by coach at 8 A.M. and arrive at Vukevar at 10. Vukevar is described as a town whose monuments were the cultural and spiritual treasures of Croatia. On the tour you will see "demolished" baroque churches, the "shattered" castle of Count Elc, the "flattened" old city. Et cetera. Et cetera. For safety reasons, you are forbidden to leave the bus and because of these "special conditions," the tour includes a packed lunch of one apéritif, soldier's beans and bread, and a liter of Riesling wine plus a doughnut.

Cost $12.40. Including an apéritif.

The next trip will be to Sarajevo. See history as it is being made.

Roger

April

Jacques Barzun is credited with having proclaimed that "whoever would know the heart and mind of America had better learn baseball." While I will never dispute that axiom, the single action that has come to epitomize much of the American character to me belonged to a figure from an entirely different and much more international sport, namely, basketball. "Red" Auerbach was for many years the coach of the most successful basketball team in the world, the Boston Celtics, who won ten championships in a single eleven-year stretch under his leadership. He was an intense competitor who fought tooth and nail, but as soon as he knew that the game was won, Red relaxed, sat back, and lit a cigar, barely watching either his team or their opponents play out the rest of the game. That act was not one of disdain or arrogance. He had won. He had no more worries. He could relax and enjoy himself. He could sit back and feel the thrill of victory. If his actions increased the agony of defeat, so be it.

April 1

Dear Rob,

I went to see my dentist yesterday. Not really my dentist but my dentist's dental hygienist, who chiseled the plaque off my teeth. It's an annual trek that I make once every two or three years. Regularly. It not only serves to clean my teeth and save my gums, but also gives me a chance to catch up on *People* and *Sports Illustrated* as I always have to wait at least half an hour. Why? I don't know. I'm sure she couldn't have had an emergency each and every day I have an appointment; yet she's always half an hour late. But I don't complain, it gives me my chance to read all those great articles.

I started with a copy of *SI*. An old issue. That didn't matter. I wasn't reading it to catch up on the latest in the NBA. I read about baseball. It makes for far better writing than football or basketball. George Plimpton thinks that is because of the size of the ball. That the quality of the writing is inversely proportional to the size of the ball, the smaller the ball the better the writing. So that the order, from worst to best, from biggest to smallest, would be basketball, football, then baseball. So far so good. Think of all those great baseball books. *The Natural, You Know Me, Al, Bingo Long, The Boys of Summer*. And then golf. The ball is smaller. So is the list of good books. And great books? Name one. Hell, even baseball umpires have written good books. Has a caddie ever done that?

It's not the size of the ball that counts, it's the nature of what happens to that ball, the nature of the game itself. I will resist the temptation to make some clever off-color analogy that would include your patients. Life is not a metaphor for baseball. The reverse, of course, goes without saying.

So I read an article about Mark Koenig, the last of the '27 Yankees. Baseball's best team ever. I used his name in *Sins*. And he's still alive. Or at least he was when the article was published. I wonder if he can sue me too. Maybe he and Marty could start a class action suit. Of course, I only said he was a shortstop, not that he was dead. The truth is a defense. It worked for the Marquis of Queensbury when Oscar Wilde sued him. Unless they sue because I used his name for profit.

Sins opened with Paul Richardson trying to remember the lineup of the '27 Yanks. Gehrig at first, Lazzeri at second, Dugan at third. Columbia Lou, Push-em-up Tony, and Jumping Joe. But who played shortstop? He could not remember. Try as he would. Then a week and

214

eight deaths later, on the last page, he remembers. Koenig—Mark Koenig.

Well, he's still alive. He ended his career playing shortstop for the '32 Cubs. They played the Yankees, those same Yankees with Leo Durocher at shortstop. That I knew. And Mark Koenig was the cause of the ill will between the two teams. Before the series, the teams each voted how to split the World Series booty. The Cubs only voted Koenig half a share. I knew that. After all, he only played half a season. The Yankees called them a bunch of cheapskates, which they were. They retaliated by calling Ruth overweight and over the hill, which he also was. Then in that classic scene Ruth shut them up. He let two strikes go by, stepped out of the batter's box, and pointed to the center field bleachers and called his shot.

One pitch. One swing. One historic home run. Into the center field bleachers. Ruth had called his shot. Did it really happen? Cynics doubt it. There are, unbelievably, no films of it. There were 31,000 fans in the stands. Conservatively speaking, at least 100,000 Chicagoans now claim to have been there and remember seeing it. No one I ever met claims to have been there and not seen it. What's that got to do with the size of the ball?

Koenig had been in the minor leagues and had been called up to replace the regular Cub shortstop, Billy Jurges. Why? Because Jurges had been shot in a hotel room by a woman. I hadn't known that. That means that Eddie Waitkus was not the only one. Did Bernard Malamud know about Billy Jurges? Did Eddie Waitkus? Size of the ball? Never. Was any basketball player shot by a female friend? Shot in the original sense of the word, not shot up with something. Somehow baseball still allows for romance, in the original sense of the word.

Roger

April 2

Dear Rob,

I've just been reading Normal Mailer's *Harlot's Ghost*. Actually I've been listening to it, not reading it. No matter. He still gets his royalties. Double. He, himself, did the recording. That's not the point. The point is that one of the CIA agents, a thoroughly despicable character, has the cover name of Randy (nice double entendre there) Huff "based on Sam Huff, the linebacker for the New York Giants." Based on. Derived from.

Is Huff suing Mailer? Is his publisher holding back his royalties? Mailer's, that is; not Huff's. Any bets? I must send a copy of this to my lawyer. I wonder what Huff does for a living. I doubt that he sells insurance.

I don't know if you've been following the troubles of artist Jeff Koons. I have. Not the obscene sculptures of him and his wife going at it in various ways. That bores me terrifically. I'll take my pornography straight, if you don't mind. It's the affair of the purloined photo that I have found interesting.

The facts. In 1980 a photographer named Art Rogers did a photograph of a couple with eight German shepherd puppies in their laps. In 1988 Koons did a sculpture called "String of Puppies" in painted wood of the same scene. Same couple. Same eight puppies. Same bench. Exact same scene.

Rogers sued for copyright infringement. In Rogers' words, Koons' sculpture was a total rip-off. "He took my photo, made it into a sculpture, and made a lot of profit on it." There is no question that Koons used Rogers' copyrighted notecard as the basis for his work. Koons called it "appropriation"; Rogers called it piracy. The court agreed with Rogers.

According to the judge, "The copying was so deliberate as to suggest that defendants resolved so long as they were significant players in the art business, and the copies they produced bettered the price of the copied works by a thousand to one, their piracy of a less well-known artist's work would escape being sullied by an accusation of plagiarism."

Foul play, cry the artists. Infringement on freedom of speech. The best comment came from another appropriation artist, Robert Yarber. He was worried that this legal discussion could result in a "resurgence of the cult of originality." I sure as hell hope it does.

Roger

April 6

Dear Rob,
  Gloom.
  Doom.
  Disaster.
  Disaster of disasters. Even a book auction without any bids would be no worse than this. Even a bad review in the *New York Times Book Review*. No, not by exaggerating. Not by much, at least. Hyperbole becomes me. The data is all in. It has all been scrutinized and analyzed. Rescrutinized. Reanalyzed. And reanalyzed again. And, believe it or not, Landau was right. Or at least righter than he had any right to be. The Oracle of St. Louis has been vindicated. Or revindicated. He claimed that the seeming effect of Eldepryl on the course of Parkinson's disease was an illusion, the result of a mild but definite therapeutic effect. We had been treating their symptoms, not their disease process. And now all the data is in and, damn it, he was probably right. Eldepryl had more of a therapeutic effect than we thought it did. We, those of us who perpetrated the pyramid scheme, or was it a Panzi scheme? I forget. Well, we were far too compulsive for our own good. We should have published our study in the *New England Journal* and called it quits. But we couldn't do that. We are scientists. There were t's that needed to be crossed and i's to be dotted. So we all went back to our respective bucket shops and continued studying all of the patients in our study. Science at work. Collecting more data to strengthen our conclusion and to silence our critics. We took special care in studying those patients who were still on Eldepryl; we took them off to see if that made much of a difference. The best way to tell if Eldepryl was having a therapeutic effect and to prove that it wasn't would be to take all the patients off their Eldepryl. If Eldepryl was making no difference, being off would make no difference. If it was making a difference, once they were off they would deteriorate, their Parkinson's disease would seem worse. And we had the perfect scale to measure that. The good old UPDRS. The Unified Parkinson's Disease Rating Scale.
  We examined each patient, filled out the UPDRS form, and then took them off Eldepryl for thirty days. Hundreds of patients on no medicine at all. We examined them again. Another UPDRS form. Garcia was never this careful. Off to the statisticians. They crunched all the numbers and, bingo, not much of a difference. Good. That's what was supposed to have happened.

But we didn't stop then, we kept them off Eldepryl and on no medicine at all for thirty more days, a total of sixty days. Hundreds of Parkinson's disease patients in bucket shops around the country being carefully followed and evaluated on no medicine at all. And at the end of sixty days another UPDRS. More data. More numbers. More crunching. And a different answer. This time they got worse. Worse than they had been on Eldepryl. Eldepryl had had a significant therapeutic effect. Just as Landau had predicted. More than we had thought it would. Was the beneficial effect sufficient to account for its protective effect?

Perhaps. But perhaps not. Possibly not. Probably not? We're not sure. Landau was, in the end, right. In substance, if not in style. And style is not everything. Back to the bucket shops. In the good ol' days, Panzi schemes were never like this.

Sell your Mylan.

Roger

April 9

Dear Rob,

So in the end are we all like good ol' Richard Wagner? Not in the lives we lead. You, I hope, wouldn't run off and have an affair with Cosima Liszt von Bulow. And father an illegitimate child. Not with the wife of a good friend and one of your most ardent champions. For that was the role von Bulow had played, friend and champion. And continued to play.

And we don't write anti-Semitic tracts. And neither of us would demand that Hermann Levi, the man we personally chose to conduct the world premiere of that most Christian of operas, *Parsifal*, convert in order to interpret the music correctly.

I didn't make any of this up. These are the facts, Rob. And we don't confuse operatic symbolism with religious ritual, or vice versa.

So how are we like Richard Wagner, if not in our personal lives, not acting out on our prejudices, but in our lives as creative artists? The answer is in the words. We have the same lack of self-judgment he did. Both as scientists and as artists. Wagner believed that his true calling was as a dramatist. That that was his great contribution to music theater, to musical dramas. The words. Not the music, the words. The story line.

218

Complete with giants and dragons, and spells, and magic fires, and potions, and gods. Gods galore. Could anyone have even taken any of that claptrap seriously?

How would you grade Wagner? Composition: A+. Lyrics: B. He was no Lorenz Hart. Nor even a Lorenzo da Ponte. Book: D. Certainly no da Ponte. Not even George S. Kaufman could have saved those librettos. Self-judgment: D+. But, and this is a big but, he sure as hell did get the music so damn right.

I can hear your disclaimer, without your having to bother to write it down. That's true of artists. They are all tied up in being artists. Creation. Imagination. Run amok. So, of course, self-judgment is not reliable. But not scientists. Science has method and rigor. And all that. So my claim is preposterous.

WRONG.

The scientific method is independent of all self-criticism. And so is peer review. What do we judge? The process. Hypothesis. Methods. Especially the methods. Data. Analysis. Statistics. Did the scientist use the right statistical method? Discussion. But not whether the experiment was really worthwhile to do in the first place.

Significance is not just a statistical question. It is a matter of judgment. Self-judgment. It isn't that most science is above that. The problem is that most science assumes that it is. Now that is real arrogance. As arrogant as picking Hermann Levi and then demanding that he convert. Why not just let von Bulow conduct and be over with it?

And Wagner is the best example of a creative genius who had no idea as to the true significance of what he was about. If he was so far off base, what hope is there for the rest of us?

So others must always act in judgment. But who? Peer review? Editors? Not medical editors. I'm talking about literature here. Publishers? Those guys who are willing to put their money on the line.

The government?

The Senate Judiciary Committee—you remember them, Rob. They're the guys who held the Clarence Thomas hearings. A group of major league ethicists, if ever there was one. Well, the Senate Judiciary Committee is at it again. This time they are considering a bill to compensate the victims of pornography. No, not the bored patrons who have to sit through those awful movies in the hope of being titillated or finding the redeeming social virtues. Virtue at the porno house. And not the actresses who have to fake all those orgasms. The faking of orgasms may be more up their alley than virtue, but certainly not a subject they would tackle face-on. So to speak. It's far more devious than that. This proposed bill would allow a victim of rape, for instance, to bring a civil suit against publishers or distributors of "obscene" or "pornographic" material if it can be proven that that material was a "substantial cause of the offense," and if the publisher or distributor should have "foreseen" that the material itself created a "reasonable risk" of such a crime being stimulated.

Don't laugh. These guys are actually considering this bill. And it's not just "these guys" who are to blame. Several feminist groups are pressuring them.

Step back. Look at the words. "Substantial cause." "Foreseen." "Reasonable risk." It would be a lawyer's fantasy come true. Another cause of action. Almost impossible to prove. Harder yet to disprove. A null hypothesis that cannot be disproven. Move over, Sigmund. You have company. Lawsuits galore. With no winners.

Then why? One reason and one reason only. Censorship. Prior censorship. That is censorship pure and simple. A scare tactic. I didn't mean to do it. But I read *Lady Chatterley's Lover*, so I raped her. She should sue the publisher. And the author, too, I'm sure. Since the author undoubtedly will have to sign a contract in which he indemnifies the publisher against such suits.

Why not include gun manufacturers? Or liquor distributors? Or drug pushers? Or physicians? A *non sequitur?* Think about it. You describe a new surgical procedure. Someone else reads your article. He performs the surgery. You obviously had foreseen that. That's why you wrote the article in the first place.

He screws up. That happens. And should have been foreseen. By you! So the patient sues you. Why not? You have more insurance.

End result: keep the procedure to yourself. That's called censorship. And that's how it works. But I'm sure the great ethicists in the senate will protect us all.

Hermann Levi, by the way, did not, I repeat, did not, convert. And he did conduct the premiere of *Parsifal*.

Did you know that Elias Lonnrot was born on this day in 1802? Admit it; you didn't. As you must recall, he was a Finnish physician who, guess what, became a writer. Before it was all the rage. After Tobias Smallett and Oliver Goldsmith, true, but long before Conan Doyle or Chekhov. After Lonnrot received his medical degree from the University of Helsinki, he became a district medical officer in a remote part of eastern Finland. Must have been some sort of national service. Like we ought to have here. I'm sure that it must be hard to get more remote than any place the Finns consider remote. While stationed there, he made medical rounds among the Lapps, the Estonians, and the Finns, collecting folktales as he went along. Ballads, poems, tales, sketches. He believed that all of the early Finnish poems he collected were fragments of a single great epic that had become lost. So he reconstructed it as he made his house calls, adding his own material to connect the parts and then constructing a plot to hold his epic together. I guess William Carlos Williams wasn't the first physician to write an epic. Lonnrot's method would certainly be frowned upon today. Not his writing lines between patients, but his inserting that writing between fragments. The result was *Kalevala*, which became the Finnish national epic.

He became professor of Finnish at the University of Helsinki and played a major role in the revival of the Finnish language and in the birth of modern Finnish literature. Before *Kalevala*, the language of literature had been Swedish. No more.

Roger

April 12

Dear Rob,

Last night I went to see a foreign film, one of those serious films, one of the ones you have to read. It reminded me of something the great American political humorist/satirist Will Rogers claimed, that he never met a man he didn't like. Will made that statement long before the era in which the Nobel Prize Committee awarded Peace Prizes to the likes of Henry Kissinger and Yassir Arafat and in one sense made the profession of political satirist obsolete or, as the British would say, "redundant." Well, I never read a motion picture [read "movie" or, better yet, "film"] that I did like. That was a conclusion that I had reached long before I became a neurologist. Since many of my friends loved such films, friends who read the same books that I did, who went to the same plays, and even some who liked the same operas, I was certain that this apparent idiosyncrasy of mine was just that, an idiosyncrasy arising out of a childhood wasted watching baseball games instead of reading great books, of thinking of books as literature and movies as entertainment.

That peculiar prejudice lasted until I saw "Bad Day at Black Rock" and realized that movies could be far more than just entertaining. It had to be me. Not the films. Not the media. Not even the message. Me. A defect of my own personality, of my upbringing, of my experience. Nurture not nature. But a nurturing process that had been so pervasive that it had become an integral part of how I acted and felt, of how I perceived the world. So be it. I've survived worse. I'm a White Sox fan!

Over the years, my own perverse response has been reinforced every time I suffered through such a film. Oh, I keep going. Or keep getting taken. I went last night. Mostly I end up reading French films. Comedies, I'm told. And I've hated them all. I disliked them as an undergraduate. As a medical student. As a resident learning about the brain, its functions, and its diseases, and finally as a full-fledged neurologist. I went to those movies with my friends and I barely tolerated them. Each and every time, I came out of the theater feeling that I had somehow been gypped. I hadn't seen a movie. And all the while I remained convinced that it was my fault.

No more. I am a changed man. I still hate such films but two things have changed. I rarely go. I have almost completely given up inflicting such torture on myself. Leave the self-flagellation to others. And, far more significantly, I now understand that my response is not my fault. Nor my parent's. Nor my beloved White Sox. It's not due to nurture. But nature. My nature. Our nature. The nature of our brains. Brains that were made to experience movies in that way. It cannot be done. Once you start reading, you can no longer see the movie. Unfortunate but true. Dubbing works. Titles don't. And anyone who thinks they do is fooling himself. It's just the way our brains evolved. *And* being able to read while seeing anything else has never been a factor in that evolution. My inability to experience the nature of a motion picture while reading subtitles is a result of how my brain functions. It is a neurologic problem, pure and simple. One we all share. Not an idiosyncrasy. A reality. Our brains were not made to read. That's too mechanistic. They did not evolve to read. No one ever said, "I read, ergo I am."

I should start at the beginning. Back with amphioxus and Darwin. Reading is not a natural part of life. It has never played a role in survival of the fittest. It is an artifact of the invention of writing. A very recent artifact at that. As such, it is an ability that is only four or five thousand years old. And, and this is the key, it is not performed by a system that evolved specifically to perform that task. Reading started full bloom on one fine day. Ergo it is performed by systems designed for something else and put to work on reading. It has no specific anatomic system of its own.

Vision does. Vision goes back to amphioxus and even before that. Visual spots and all that. So does hearing. And hearing allows for parallel perception. Correction. In the survival of the fittest, a hearing system was perfected that included parallel perception. Take a Gershwin song. You can hear the words [Ira's] and the music [George's] simultaneously. Why? Survival value. Animals listen for the sound of what they are pursuing and yet still attend to the sound that might be pursuing them. Parallel perception.

None of this applies to reading. Vision, yes. Reading, no. Reading is not just vision. The visual image of the written word is not processed by that part of the brain that recognizes visual images. The man who mistook his wife for a hat could still read. The images of words get shunted off to the speech areas. Not a place where visual images go in any other species. Nor in nonliterate humans.

How did it then come about? Not by random variation, struggle to survive, and survival of the fittest. That was not Darwin's term. That phrase was coined by Spenser. It is the result of learned appropriation, an effort that must be relearned by each generation, and not without effort. An effort that requires our complete attention. We can talk and listen and do so many things with parallel perception paralleling away. But not so reading. The attention that it requires diverts all of our attention. Reading aborts parallel perception.

The result is that you can't see a movie if you are reading it. You can listen to the words and hear the music and see the action. That's what our brains were designed to do. So to speak. But if you are reading the words, you can't really see the movie, not in the way it was meant to be seen. It wasn't my fault at all. It's reality. I had always been right to hate reading movies. I just didn't understand why. Now I do. Ain't neurology great? It gives a scientific basis to our prejudices.

My original conclusion about reading movies was also far removed from the time in which I began to take myself seriously as a writer. Now I even worry about the structure of Will's statement. Did he not mean that he came to like everyone he met? Ergo he liked everyone he met. Not he met everyone he already liked before they were even introduced to him. So much for language. I take myself more seriously as a scientist.

Roger

April 14

Dear Rob,

This is my one hundredth letter to you. Number 100. 1-0-0. I know it seems like more than that. So go ahead. Count them. I'll wait. . . . That's right; you don't have to count them again.

So how did I come up with one hundred? The editors. They are bound to delete some, combine others. Switch the order. And in so doing change the total number that I have written. Not the number you have read, but the precise number that actually have an existence. So it is now one hundred. A perfect denominator.

Don't worry. I will not emulate Charles Dodgson. A man of many talents. Far better known as Lewis Carroll. Mathematician of the first order. A don, whatever that is, at Oxford. A deacon of the Church of England. An intense amateur photographer. I almost wrote pornographer. Those photographs he took of the naked Alice Lidell are more than mere photographs. They would certainly fall under today's laws against child pornography. They have long been considered "delicately erotic." Well, her mother was right. She refused Dodgson access to the house and her daughter.

Back to my letters. My one hundred letters. Dodgson, between his other tasks, photographic and nonphotographic, managed somehow to write over one hundred thousand letters. That does not count the letters he wrote to Alice Lidell. Her mother burned them. Our loss? Posterity's? Or the right act by a mother protecting her daughter?

There's a good question for you. I'm on the mother's side.

One hundred thousand letters, all written in thirty-six years. That's two thousand seven hundred and seventy-eight letters per year, a little over seven and a half letters a day. With no word processor. And no telephone. There's the key. He had to write letters. Seven and a half letters a day seems astronomical to us. But many of them are no more than brief phone calls in writing. And no more worth preserving.

Calls to his publisher. To his illustrator. His editor. His relatives. As phone calls they would have no independent existence, which is as it should be. But letters do. And should. Some have now been published. *The Looking Glass Letters.* Had he just made dirty phone calls to all those little girls such a book could never exist.

My first copy of *Acumen* arrived today. I read it. So did *Neurology.* Ditto. More or less. One of the articles was by Anna Adams. She's a poet,

I presume. Her article, of course, appeared in *Acumen*, not *Neurology*. I suppose if she read one of my articles, she'd presume I was a scientist. So be it. *Caveat emptor*. "Poetry Parasite" was the title of her piece. It was an essay, not a poem. It was all about criticism. The criticism of poetry. Not a subject I'd ever read very much about. What's wrong with poetry today, she wrote, is that the poets and critics are all the same people. Peer criticism, in the truest sense. This to her is a grievous error. But that is what is supposed to be right about science. Of the few things we scientists do right. It's called peer review.

Anna Adams does not think that this process is a good thing. Just the opposite. It results in a closed world for both poetry and science. A self-propagating and self-satisfied closed world made up of self-aggrandizing parts. She does have a point there.

But that is not all. She also pointed out that "too much average poetry is not a healthy diet for a poet." Could she also be right about that? For both poetry and science? Could too much average science not be a healthy diet for a scientist? Too much mediocre science? Mediocre is not used in any pejorative sense, just in its real sense. Its real meaning. Humdrum. Average.

Most of what I read on the average is mediocre at best.

She then went on to add that newspapers and books about science are more nourishing and useful for the poet than mediocre poems. Could poetry books be more useful for the scientist?

I am always refreshed when an article makes me think. I just wish more of them came from *Neurology* than *Acumen*. Or do I?

Roger

April 20

Dear Rob,

We hosted our second implant meeting this weekend. Isn't it amazing the number of things I do that you don't know about until they are over, the number of letters I send out without copying you. Be glad. Most of them are boring. That includes both categories. The meeting itself was not. In format it was pretty much like the first one, the one held in early December. Once again we tried to invite all of the investigators interested in doing implants on Parkinson's disease patients and everybody got an equal shot at the podium. Not a free-for-all, but equal opportunity on a tight schedule. Several research groups reported partial benefits following adrenal implants, very similar to our results. In fact, the similarity of the observations was striking. The patients all followed the same time course. No one got better immediately. Then the patients slowly began to improve. Not get cured, but get better. How much better? Not as much as they wanted to or as much as we wanted them to, but there is no denying it, something is going on. Those implants are obviously having a beneficial effect. That is evident. But enough to be worth all the risk?

Garcia had been invited and he had promised to come. We were all anxious and waiting. The meeting started on Friday. No Garcia.

On Saturday there was still no Garcia but there was a telegram, a message from Garcia, so to speak. He would arrive in time to speak on Sunday. Could we give him an hour? No one else had been given more than twenty minutes, but I juggled the schedule. He is the reason we're doing all of this.

Then on Sunday morning, Garcia arrived direct from Spain, where he'd been hailed at the meeting of Spanish neurologists. He presented his summary of what he had accomplished. He told us about his thirty-five patients. Thirty-five! An impressive total. As many as the three or four most active U.S. groups combined. Twice as many as we knew about before.

But nagging questions remained. At least for many of us. Was that all? Was that the entire number? Was he making a full disclosure this time? I had my doubts. And, believe me, Rob, I was not alone. Were our doubts justified?

Garcia assured us that he was telling it all. Telling it like it was. We were all willing to accept that. We were not an easy audience, but we wanted him to be right. We were invested in that. Not as invested as he was, but invested none the less. We'd bet on him. We were doing his procedure on our own patients. Sure, many of us were still skeptical. How could we be otherwise? We'd been burned once. But this had to be different.

After describing his procedure, he got on to the results. All of his patients were "greatly improved." I stopped him. I wanted to make certain that we had all heard him correctly. Had he said that all of his patients were "greatly improved?"

He had.

All? One hundred percent?

All, he reiterated.

That question and answer were repeated several more times. He meant what he'd said. Each and every patient was greatly improved.

He then expanded upon his results. Not only were the patients improved as far as their Parkinson's disease, that was only the beginning; they were "junger," he said. "Much junger."

"Junger," I repeated to myself. "Junger?"

What the hell was he talking about?

Junger? Like the analyst? Jung. That Nazi.

No. He didn't mean that. It wasn't Jung. It was young. He meant that they were younger. His patients were younger. No. That was impossible. It must be a problem in linguistics.

"You mean they look younger?" I asked, hoping to clear the air of the resentment that I could feel building up.

"No. Not look. They are. They are all junger."

My God, I thought, he really believes it. It's not linguistics. It was a far deeper difference. I was certain at that moment that he actually believed that his patients had become younger. Ponce de Leon reborn. A successful Ponce de Leon. It was as if he were a used car salesman who believed what he said. Every single word of it. And we'd all bought a car from him.

From there, the conference just deteriorated. Physicians from around the country asked Garcia about specific patients on whom he'd operated. Patients they had seen, the physician from Pennsylvania. The one who had come to see us.

"His Parkinson's is better," Garcia told us all. "He is better." His operation a success. Shades of Margaret Bourke White. He got so much better he could no longer practice medicine or live by himself or take care of himself. I always thought that success was made of sterner stuff. Or at least better data.

Then he was asked about a woman from California.

Did he remember her?

He did.

And her surgery?

A success.

The doctor who asked about her had been treating her for years. He still was. Did Dr. Garcia realize that she had been in a chronic vegetative state since the surgery? That she was now in a nursing home? Immobile! All but in a coma. There was nothing she could do for herself. She could not walk or talk. Or feed herself.

"Yes, but her Parkinson's is better."

Could he really believe that? He said it. I heard it. So did all the others who were there. But this woman was in a nursing home unable to speak or move. Not even a used car salesman could really believe that. Was she, too, younger?

He then went on to describe his experiments in rats. They, too, were younger. Ponce De Leon extending his kingdom.

Who cared?

Not I.

Suddenly I got a bad feeling in the pit of my stomach. What had happened to Fred Gould? He had gone to Mexico. That had been about a couple of months ago. I hadn't heard from him since.

Nothing strange about that. He was not really my patient. We'd turned him down. We'd refused to operate on him. That's why he'd gone to Mexico City.

I asked Garcia.

"He is much better," I was told. Somehow I was not reassured by that reply.

As soon as I could get away, I called Geneva. A man answered. A man named Michel Adler, a friend of Fred's. He knew who I was.

"Can I speak to Fred?" I asked.

I couldn't.

"Why not?"

"Because, Professor, Fred cannot speak. He had a stroke in Mexico City."

"When?"

"Right after the surgery?"

"Can he walk?"

"He can hardly swallow."

228

So, he, too, was much better and probably also "junger." And he only went there because of me. In more ways than one.

Roger

April 23

Dear Rob,

We held our auction today. You remember the auction. *The Blind Observer*. My AIDS novel. The triumphant return of Paul Richardson, né Richards. We held our auction and no one came. No one showed up. It was worse than an old White Sox-St. Louis Browns game. There weren't even any hotdog vendors. And more importantly, no players. You got it. We didn't get a single bid for the book. Zero for nineteen. Like Willie Mays. His major league career started that way. He went hitless for a week. Zero for twenty-three, I think. And now he's in the Hall of Fame.

I guess it's time to retire *The Blind Observer* and recalculate my batting average. I am now three for eight. That comes out to .375. Higher than Willie Mays' lifetime average. Still higher than Ty Cobb's. He still has the highest lifetime batting average. .367.

No one wanted to publish a novel, a mystery about AIDS. It didn't fit on anyone's list. That's what they all said to my agent. No one wants to read about AIDS in a mystery. A mystery is to escape from reality, not to confront it. A mystery can confront murder, drugs, rape, incest, as long as it's someone else's incest. AIDS is a taboo subject. Not mainline. Not escapist.

Why didn't my agent say that to me last year when I outlined the idea to him? He's the one who is supposed to know about publishing. I know about neurology and he knows about the publishing world. He doesn't tell me how to practice neurology and I don't tell him how to sell books, but why didn't he warn me? Why didn't he tell me before I wrote that damn book that it would be a hard sell? Isn't that his job?

I'd think so. Preventive agenting. Like preventive neurology. An ounce of prevention. A couple of words. But he didn't say anything. He said it was a great idea, brilliant, a sure sell. Just like he always says.

Maybe I need a new agent. Instead of feeling like a player who just struck out for the twenty-third time, I can pretend I own the whole team. And my team just lost for the twenty-third time. I'll do just what any owner would do. Fire the manager. Hire a new one. I'll find a new agent.

I won't have any trouble. I have a great track record. Book-of-the-Month Club. Literary Guild. And a great batting average. 1.000. What he doesn't know won't hurt him. This is publishing. Show biz. Not science. Not medicine. Garcia said he was two for two. Two miracles out of two. 1.000. Not two for ten. .200. And I castigate him. And now I'll tell a new agent that I'm three for three.

Am I any different? Hell, no. It's the words that are different.

Caveat agentor. There's no need for informed consent. Nor truth in any form. No matter what I tell an agent, none of them will believe it's the truth. If I say three for three, they'll assume it's three for six. Why should they assume I'm giving them real numbers? That's not within their realm of experience.

And that's the difference. I may quibble about the interpretation of some data I read in an *NEJM* article, but I assume the data is real. That two out of two is two out of two, not two out of three. Those are different.

Significantly so. No, just statistically so. After going zero for twenty-three, Willie Mays hit a home run. Off of Warren Spahn. Hall of Fame left-hander. The winningest pitcher since World War Two. Spahn, Sain, and pray for rain. And Willie's first home run came off of him. There may be some hope.

Roger

April 27

Dear Rob,

I have a perfect plot for you. I will not use it because I am already working on this book. And, like so many good plots, it is a true story. So first the story. The source was a lawyer, a lawyer who specializes in medical malpractice and is a friend of mine. You should be neither surprised nor scandalized, my friend. He wanted my advice on a possible cause of action. The patient was a woman in her mid-thirties who had been treated for a number of years for myasthenia gravis and finally had surgery to remove her thymus gland. During the surgery something went wrong and now she is in a permanent coma.

When you were an intern we didn't know very much about myasthenia. Today we know a lot more. Myasthenia is associated with severe fatigue and muscle weakness. That hasn't changed, but now we know what causes weakness. The thymus gland produces T cells. That's what the thymus gland does. The T cells make antibodies, which is their job. But in myasthenia, these T cells make antibodies that cause the weakness. The treatment now is to take out the thymus gland. No more new T cells. No more new antibodies. The old T cells die off. The old antibodies break down with time. No more myasthenia. No more fatigue.

I was not impressed. Things always went wrong during surgery.

"But she didn't have myasthenia," he protested.

That was his case. If she hadn't had myasthenia, then the surgery was not indicated and whatever went wrong should never have had the chance to go wrong.

"How do you know that?" I inquired.

"Her antibody level is now normal."

"That's what the surgery is supposed to do," I educated him. "The Garden Tomb," I added.

"What's that?"

"It's in Jerusalem. In the 1880s or '90s, the famous British General Chinese Gordon went to Jerusalem. He was certain that the Church of the Holy Sepulcher was in the wrong place. Jews always buried their dead outside the city walls. Golgotha was outside the city. The Church of the Holy Sepulcher is within the walls. No matter that those are different walls.

"So he went looking. He found a hill that with enough imagination and at the right angle, with the light just right, looked like a skull. And Golgotha, if you remember your Greek."

"What Greek?"

I went on, "Golgotha means skull. Calvary. Calvarium. Skull. So he started to dig and he found a first century Jewish grave."

"So?"

"It was empty," I explained.

"So?"

"That is the one thing that is known about the Holy Sepulcher."

"What's that?"

"Jesus is not in it. It is empty."

"What's that got to do with my case?"

"The fact that she doesn't have myasthenia now doesn't mean she never had. The antibodies are supposed to be gone. Normal. Their being gone now cannot tell us anything about what they were before. About who was in that grave."

"She didn't have it."

"I'm sure her antibodies were high."

"Never measured pre-op. It was a clinical diagnosis based on history and examination."

"Like a real doctor. That's what we all used to do."

"Four years ago?"

"No," I admitted, but that still wasn't malpractice and there was no way for me to prove that she hadn't had myasthenia. No way at all.

"Myasthenia is rare, isn't it?"

"Yes."

"How rare?"

"One case in fifty thousand a year."

"She lives in Joliet. That's about fifty thousand. That year her doctor diagnosed thirty cases, and operated on them all and. . . ."

"Now all their graves are empty."

"You guessed it."

"A class action suit," I suggested. "It was a good scam he had. Diagnose a disease and then cure it."

And that, my friend, is the kernel of the plot. To make it sexier, you merely change the disease. HIV. AIDS. Bogus test results of wealthy clients followed by some mysterious and, of course, expensive experimental cure. It's a start. And the plot's the easy part, my boy.

David has me reading Siegfried Sassoon's diaries. It is not just letters that create a legacy. So do literary diaries. And notebooks. Gide. Camus. Auden. Sassoon. Sassoon's diary is populated by famous people, significant others in both senses. Robert Graves, before *I, Claudius* was in.

H.G. Wells a.k.a. just plain old H. G. The two Lawrences, D.H. and T.E. [Lawrence of Arabia]. More T.E. than D.H. Thomas Hardy. E.M. Forster, before everything he wrote was in. Henry Head. Head was a neurologist. One of the greats of his era. An expert on aphasia. Editor of *Brain*. I'm not making this up. Head edited *Brain* and was succeeded by Russell Brain. S.S. went to see *Tristan*, but he intentionally missed an entire act. Missing an act, he wrote, always increased his enjoyment of Wagner. There may be much more to Sassoon than I had thought.

Roger

April 29

Dear Rob,

Oliver Messiaen died yesterday. In France. He was 83. I heard about it this morning while listening to WFMT as I was driving in to the hospital. No, you should not have heard of him. And, yes, you should have. It all depends on whether or not you have a serious interest in contemporary classical music. For he was a composer of very serious contemporary classical music. WFMT is our premiere classical music station. They played some of his music this morning. His *Quartet for the End of Time*. He composed it in 1941, the announcer said.

I knew that.

While he was interned in Stalag 8A. I didn't know that. I didn't know that this piece had been composed in a concentration camp. Hell, I didn't even know that Messiaen had been in a Nazi concentration camp.

Why? Why had he been interned? Concentrated, so to speak. He wasn't Jewish. He was a devout Catholic. Almost all of his music is basically religious. Sort of like Bach, only more so. Messiaen composed religious music because that was the need he felt, not because it was his job. Or he had a commission to do so.

Max Jacob, I remembered, was also a devout Catholic. He had been one since he had converted in 1909. A conversion that was prompted by a vision of Jesus that appeared on the wall of his studio. Not the Shroud of Turin, but good enough for Max. Max had converted. He had been born a Jew. To the Nazis, being a Jew was not a matter of religion. Religions, after all, come and go. It was a matter of genes.

233

Max was a Jew. Forever. So in 1944 he was arrested. Interned. Concentrated.

But Messiaen had not been born a Jew. Had he been a leftist? I always thought of him as rather withdrawn and ascetic. Not as a political activist. Not as an agitator. Had he been a communist in his youth? And had a later conversion? Had he been in the Underground? Or had he merely been in the wrong place at the wrong time?

He was in Stalag 8A. While Birkmayer, my old friend, was in the SS. Birkmayer was Jewish. Not according to religion. Or tradition. Or any Rabbi. But according to the SS.

And in 1944 they arrested Max Jacob.

Jean Cocteau was horrified. Jacob was a great man of letters. The man who had invented the French prose poem. The poet who had written surrealist poetry before Tzara invented the word Dada and before Breton, that physician turned writer, discovered surrealism. Before de Chirico even. And Jacob had friends. Picasso. So many others.

Cocteau wrote a petition. He got everyone to sign it. The Germans must free Max Jacob. He was a member of the Legion of Honor. How French could you get? How Catholic? Almost everyone signed the petition. Almost. But not all. Not Picasso. Picasso refused. No one ever accused Picasso of loyalty to old friends. Or of being a great humanist.

Jacob was packed into a cattle car and died en route to oblivion. Of pneumonia. The old man's best friend. In 1944. He was sixty-eight.

One of the problems of wanting to be taken seriously is that it might happen. If it does, your actions become significant. And your non-actions. They, too, have a meaning. A meaning that pervades your work.

The ever-flippant Jean Cocteau wrote a petition.

The ever-significant Pablo Picasso refused to sign it.

Yes, Picasso painted *Guernica*. And Cocteau is seen as a gadfly of sorts. A dilettante in the best sense of that word. More an Ogden Nash or a James Thurber than a William Faulkner. Not quite to be taken seriously.

WFMT also played some Beethoven and some Brahms conducted by Sir Thomas Beecham. Beecham had been born on this day one hundred and thirteen years ago. And they could only pay tribute to him because of those recording engineers he so hated. The horns, I trust, were not too loud.

R.I.P.

Roger

234

May

When the police arrived at the garage on Clark Street where the St. Valentine's Day's Massacre had just taken place, one of the victims was still alive. He was Frank Gusenberg, one of the last remaining members of the then all but extinct Bugs Moran gang.

"Who shot you?" the cops asked.

"Nobody shot me," Frank informed them.

Harold L. Klawans
Newton's Madness

May 1

Dear Rob,

I was quoted in *Science* this week. That has got to be almost as important as writing a book review for the *New York Times Book Review*. Not as important as being reviewed there. That's more like publishing an article in *Science*. I've never done that. I tried once. And my article was rejected. It was later published elsewhere. Where? I'll never tell. I've been published in *NEJM*. More than once. Four times, in fact. With a batting average of four out of five. .800. I never said I needed a new agent for my scientific ventures.

Science published a report on the implant meeting we hosted. The *NEJM*, by the way, didn't. One cannot expect miracles. You may find it hard to believe but I came off as a master of understatement. Can you imagine that? Maybe I've matured over the years. I certainly have not grown "junger."

"The American results," I said, "were clearly not as spectacular as people thought they would be." How is that for a piece of understatement? I even added that the disparity between what we were seeing in the American patients and what we had been told about the Mexican patients was "substantial." Substantial! How about overwhelming? I didn't mention the patients being "junger." Or anything about the various confrontations. That was just between us scientists.

We did our last implant this week. Number twelve. We are out of that business now. We will follow our twelve patients as carefully as possible. And present the results from time to time, but our project is closed. Maybe we'll send the results in to *Science*. Or the *NEJM*. Probably the latter.

The next rage will be fetal implants. Watch your newspapers. And the *NEJM*. Why fetal implants? Because you can get the right cells from a fetus. The cells of the substantia nigra. The ones that have died off in Parkinson's disease. The ones that really do make dopamine, ones that really ought to be able to live in the brain and make dopamine.

Will they work?

That's what research is all about, isn't it?

One of my associates asked me an interesting question today. It was about a patient she'd seen with a rather rare neurologic disorder. One that suggested to me that the lower spinal cord has a different organization from that of the upper or cervical cord. We are taught that the function of the cord consists of the ability to carry out orders and relay sensory inputs and generate simple reflexes. That's it. If part of the cord has a more complex intersegmental organization in man, we would teleologically assign this to the cervical cord on the basis of man's prehensile thumb among other upper extremity abilities. But my thesis is just the opposite. The disorder is called "painful foot-moving toes syndrome" and consists of just that.

Patient: Doctor, my foot is painful and my toes move and no one knows what's wrong.

Neurologist: I know what you have.

Patient: What do I have?

Neurologist: Painful foot-moving toes syndrome.

This rare disorder is a result of prior injury to a nerve of the leg and the movements are organized at the spinal level.

And painful hand-moving fingers syndrome does not exist. Why not?

That was the question. Why not? Injuries to the nerves of the arm are no less common than injuries to the nerves of the leg. That had to mean that the cord must be organized differently in the lumbosacral enlargement than the cervical enlargement and must have a more complex organization in the former than human neuroanatomists have yet to demonstrate (or look for). Now why would that be, I asked rhetorically. Because the dinosaur had two sets of brains. That's a line from a poem I learned before I was ten. A poem that I remember. I have no idea who wrote it. I only remember a few lines.

> You will observe from these remains,
> The creature had two sets of brains.
> One in the head, the usual place.
> And the other in the spinal base.

So the lower cord has a remnant of this old spinal cord organization and the upper cord doesn't. Ergo painful foot-moving toes syndrome.

But who wrote the poem?

Roger

May 4

Dear Rob,

You are one hundred percent correct, observation is one of the key skills that is shared by good physicians and good writers. Not by all physicians, far from it, and obviously not by all writers either. Equally far from it. But what exactly is observation? Is it the ability to see more than others or the ability to better understand what has already been seen? To give meaning to the observation that has already been made? Something beyond mere perception, a perception that includes interpretation. It is a talent that was shared by William Osler, said to be the greatest clinician of the English-speaking world of the late nineteenth and early twentieth centuries, and Charles Dickens, who needs no introduction. It was Dickens who observed and described the relationship between extreme obesity and an abnormal daytime sleepiness long before any physician. And it was Osler who validated Dickens' observation, as well as his clinical acumen, and said we should call it Pickwick's syndrome. After Dickens. To honor Dickens. And, yes, we try to teach observation to every single medical student, from day one until the day he finishes his residency. Or hers. Observation and reasoning based on those observations. New observations based on old ones. Turning the slightly bent posture of an old man into Parkinson's disease with its shuffling gait and a paucity of blinking. That bent old man is no longer just an old man. He's an old man with a simian posture. An old man with a reptilian stare. An old man with a disease that someone had the sense to see, observe, and understand. Before Parkinson, an old man, but never again.

Lub and dub have also changed over the years. From out of nowhere comes the opening snap of mitral stenosis, the soft whoosh of aortic insufficiency. That was first heard by Austin Flint. In the 1840s he was the first professor of medicine here at Rush Medical College and he was also a great observer. He heard that murmur, which now carries his name. He heard it before anyone else. Like Parkinson, he, too, observed and understood and so became an eponym. The reward for a new observation, for inventing something new for others to observe. When I wrote my first novel, I named the medical school after Austin Flint. Chicago's first great physician. I thought it was fitting. Such men should be honored.

The rest of us are not such innovative observers. We've been trained to see what others have already seen. That's not the ultimate in real observation, not in the sense of a Charles Dickens or a William Faulkner.

Or an Austin Flint. They observed what others only saw. We do not teach the ability to make those kinds of observations. That may not be a skill that can really be taught. Honed a bit, yes. Refined, yes. Oriented, absolutely. But taught, created *de novo*, probably not. What we teach is seeing. Looking and seeing. Seeing what has been seen and understanding it, but seeing what has never been seen before. Hearing that which has not been heard. And that's a hell of a lot different.

No one taught Shakespeare to be Shakespeare. Nor Osler to be Osler. Nor Dickens to be Dickens. People taught Shakespeare about the stage and its needs and conventions but not how to be Shakespeare. There has always been a lot of drivel about who was Shakespeare. It couldn't have been that guy from Stratford-upon-Avon. He never went to college. He attended no university. It had to be someone else. Sir Francis Bacon. Marlowe. Some educated man.

I never fell for that. People have been going to colleges and universities for centuries. Millions of people. Did any one of them become a second Shakespeare?

That's why I believe in eponyms. So did Charcot. He named Parkinson's disease Parkinson's disease. Parkinson had called it the "shaking palsy." Charcot felt such men should be honored. Parkinson. Duchenne. Austin Flint.

Dickens once lectured here in Chicago. So did Oscar Wilde. Why? Why did they travel here? Why does ex-NBA star forward MacAdoo still play basketball in Italy? Same reason. Because that's where the money is.

When Wilde visited Chicago, the press ignored him. Why? John L. Sullivan, the heavyweight boxing champion of the world, was in town that day. Sullivan made the front page. Wilde got no coverage at all. The world has changed less than we think in the last one hundred years.

Rob, you should stop moaning and groaning about your life as a physician. All professions have their drawbacks. That's what Johnson told Boswell. Most of ours have to do with paperwork and acronyms. And both of these come from a government dedicated to paying us less. So what? Is that why you became a physician? To make more money than you would have as a basic chemist?

You still do. Believe me. A lot more. An engineer? A physicist? A lawyer?

Well, you do. If you don't believe me, look at the statistics. And even if you make ten percent less, you still will. Or even twenty percent. Want to know what the average writer makes? Believe me, you don't.

Roger

May 5

Dear Rob,

Long Day's Journey into Night. Your mere mention of the title itself conjures up images of somnolence. My own version of a Pickwickian syndrome immediately struck me. Hypersomnolence. Uncontrollable. Where is that sleep lab of yours? Of course you slept through half of it. How could you not? The wonder is that you didn't sleep through more than just half. Or do you have insomnia?

It is far too long. It is far too self-indulgent. Way far. It is boring. The great Eugene O'Neill, our only playwright who ever received the Nobel Prize in literature. He sure forgot a lot in this one. He totally disregarded one major tenet of theater. Theater takes place in real time. A speech that takes five minutes takes five whole minutes. It cannot be speed-read. There's no skimming in the theater. No scanning. Only listening. In real time. Word for word. Did the Nobel Prize Committee see his plays? Or read them? Of course. To what did they compare them? Strindberg! Now there is food for thought.

It needs editing. Paring down. Way down. But it must be taken seriously. The problem is not that the literary establishment takes it seriously; more as a testament than as good theater, but that very same establishment fails to take *You Can't Take It With You* seriously. How many Ph.D. theses have been written on the use of doorways in Kaufman and Hart? Or any other aspect?

The French take Molière seriously, but do we do the same for George S. Kaufman? Most of the literary establishment thinks Moss Hart doubled as Rodgers' lyricist—another occupation no one takes very seriously. Did they even try to write internal rhyme schemes? I'll bet not.

I've done some reading about Messiaen. Messiaen had been in the French army. He had been a medical auxiliary. A medic of some sort. When the shooting war broke out between Germany and France, he was at Verdun. In no time at all, France crumbled into defeat and he fled toward Nancy. He and several other musicians were captured and interned in Stalag 8A in Silesia. Interned! How is that for a euphemism? You and I interned together. We interned. They were put in a damned German concentration camp for French POWs.

It was there that he wrote his *Quartet for the End of Time.* The selection of instruments was determined by the skills of his companions. One violinist, one clarinetist, one cellist, and a pianist. Messiaen himself was the pianist. They often practiced in the washroom. The piece was performed at Stalag 8A on January 15, 1941. During World War I, the great Belgian historian Henri Pirrenne had been similarly "interned." And he gave a series of lectures that were copied down and became his *History of Europe from the Fall of Rome to 1815*. And we think we struggle in trying to squeeze out a book between patients. Poor struggling us.

Today, by the way, was an anniversary. Don't be ashamed that you missed it. Be ashamed of it. It was the anniversary of the arrest in Italy of Ezra Pound, arrested for aiding and abetting the enemy during war. That simple crime is known as treason. Giving comfort and succor to the enemy, which he sure as hell did. PBS, please their souls, interviewed the arresting officer, a man named Ted Pierce. He's still alive and living in Virginia. He recognized Pound and knew that he was one of the most important poets of the twentieth century. Having heard Pound's broadcasts, he also knew that Pound had been a collaborator, a traitor. He described the suicide precautions they took. Pound was clearly depressed. Second floor room. Constant monitoring. No sharp objects. No ropes. Then Pound was transferred to Pisa on his way to Washington, where his psychiatrists protected him from ever having to face any charges, and eventually Pound was declared sane and returned to Italy a free man. The interviewer asked Ted Pierce whether in view of what followed he would do it differently if he had it to do over again. Pierce paused. Pound was a great poet. A genius. He helped Eliot create what we consider to be some of the most important poems of this or any other century. Hemingway. If he had it to do over. . . . He would place Pound on the top floor, open the windows, give him ten feet of rope, and ignore him. An honest man. With honest emotion and a true sense of justice. More honest than Pound's shrinks. More moral than William Carlos Williams, the father of us all, the one we are supposed to honor and love. Williams visited Pound in Washington. Many times, to talk poetry and stuff. How about gas chambers and that sort of thing? Or wasn't that literary enough for them? For each Fascist who died in the war, Pound had said, a hundred Yids should be lined up and shot. How's that for pure poetry? Right up there with Shakespeare and all those other Greeks.

Roger

May 8

Dear Rob,

Free association. Stream of consciousness. James Joyce. Virginia Woolf. Edvard Grieg. He started this one. Call it coincidence. Or whatever you wish. As I was driving to the hospital this morning, I tired of public radio. Some of it is tiring. So I switched to one of our two classical music stations. They were playing Grieg. *Peer Gynt*. What else? Incidental music to a play by Ibsen. In my play, my Ibsen play, one of the characters tells Ibsen that he'd never heard of his play about Peer Gynt. No one had. The music, yes. Had Ibsen set some incidental words to the music? To Grieg's immortal music?

Like Goethe to Beethoven's *Egmont*. Or was that Schiller? Does it even matter? No one reads either of them today.

Ibsen lived for a while in Dresden. So did Dostoevski. At the same time. Two of the major progenitors of modern literature in the same small city at the same time. The year was 1868. It was like John L. Sullivan and Oscar Wilde being in Chicago at the same time except that Ibsen and Dostoevski were a lot more than temporary visitors to Dresden. They both lived there and they had far more in common.

Did they ever meet? Dostoevski and Ibsen, that is. Not Sullivan and Wilde. Not that we know. Dostoevski was there as a refugee from both his creditors and the authorities. He was writing *The Possessed*. Ibsen was there as an intentional expatriate. Like Hemingway in Paris, surrounding himself with other expatriates.

Peer Gynt was behind Ibsen. So was his other poetic masterpiece, *Brand*. He was about to give birth to modern drama, to naturalism, to transform our entire concept of theater. It is because of him that no one cares who wrote *Egmont*. It is no longer a play that can be performed. Nor who wrote *Peer Gynt*.

Ibsen pulled off a revolution. And succeeded. And not just one. From romanticism to naturalism then to expressionism and modernism. *Brand* to *Hedda Gabler* to *The Master Builder*.

They never met, Dostoevski and Ibsen. What if they had? Would the course of modern literature have changed? Would *The Possessed* have been any different? Would *Hedda Gabler*? Would it, like *The Brothers Karamazov*, have been a tale about murder? Like my still unproduced version. Or would their individual visions have remained individual? The answer is obvious. Each man had his own dream.

Herzl and Freud lived on the same street in Vienna and never met. Herzl had a dream. Freud dealt with dreams. Would the world be different if they'd met? Freud asks that question in my Anna O. play. Schnitzler reminds Freud that Herzl's dream was of a different sort. Freud, my Freud, Anna's Freud, is not convinced.

Lenin, Joyce, and Tristam Tzara were all in Zurich at the same time. That was in 1916. Did they ever meet? Only in Stoppard's play *Travesties*. And there are limits to imagination and cleverness. They do not change history.

T.S. Eliot grew up on the banks of the Mississippi River. Like Huck Finn. A couple of decades later, but they could have met. Old Huck and young T.S. How's that for a scenario? A play? Isn't that what theater is all about? Getting two interesting people together who have something to say and letting them say it.

Who is more interesting, as a pair, than Huck Finn and T.S. Eliot? The idea is free. Use it as you wish. Or you could try Oscar Wilde and John L. Sullivan meeting in an Irish bar in Chicago—with one of them picking up the other. Which one? Your pick.

Roger

Hedda! A play in two acts—script still available on request.

May 10

Dear Rob,

Thank God for good ol' Jesse Helms. He and others of his ilk almost justify what we do. More and more often these days I ask myself why I still write reading. Not why I write. That question is far too basic to be asked. That answer can only be found deep within my soul. Even after that exhaustive four hour analysis, did Freud know why Mahler composed music? Why symphonies, not quartets? Why lieder and not ballets? Freud might have had enough data to hypothesize about Mahler's choice of melodies, his juxtapositions of the banal and the sublime, but not the real issue. So not why do I write, but why do I write the written word? Words meant to be read. Essays. Short stories. Novels. And why do you want to write such sentences, sentences designed to be read? Not seen. Not heard. Read. Written sentences are no longer what they once were. To say nothing of entire paragraphs. Much less complete stories.

It didn't used to be like that. *Les Miserables* caused riots. It stirred men's souls. Now it's a series of songs. But there was a time when novels changed, if not history, at least attitudes. *Uncle Tom's Cabin.* And that wasn't even literature.

So did opera. Verdi's *Nabucco.* The opera that made his career. The chorus of the Hebrew slaves became the anthem of the Italians, who felt themselves to be the slaves of the Austrians. It became their "fight" song. Verdi became a national hero. Can you imagine that today? Or censors making him change the libretto to *Un Ballo*, fearing the outcome if he didn't? Who cares about an opera libretto today?

Or a ballet? There were riots at the premiere of *The Rite of Spring* in Paris in 1914. Paris. On the eve of the Great War. And ballet was that important. The Stravinsky music. Saint Saens walked out. The Nijinsky choreography. Obscure. A scandal. Riots in the aisles. And we don't even have the real choreography. Why not? Film existed. Why was it never filmed? Never recorded for posterity? Posterity, after all, was just around the corner.

But think about it, about the riot. The music mattered. It really mattered. And the entire production. Art. Art mattered.

Today what could have that kind of effect? A new symphony? A new ballet. A new opera. Think about that. An opera. Certainly not Menotti. Philip Glass. Maybe, but not to that degree. Could an opera, any opera, cause riots in the streets? Could an opera cause anything other than disregard? Neglect. Boredom. Let's get serious.

Could art do that? Any form of art? Painting? Sculpture? You take your pick. No chance.

TV? TV and the movies? That's it.

And they have abrogated their responsibility. They reach the public. The words written for TV are heard. Those for the movies are heard. By hundreds of millions, all over the world. But so what? They are words without substance. Words to sell popcorn. And cars. Words as entertainment. Entertainment *über alles.* So to speak.

So thank God for Jesse Helms. He reminds us that art is important. It means something. It means everything. It counts. If art didn't count, who would care? Certainly not Senator Jesse Helms. Art matters. It sways men's minds. What a concept. What a belief. Right on, Jesse. Art matters. Literature matters. Not the latest made-for-TV movie. Those censor themselves of all real content.

I've written a treatment on Jack Kevorkian and his mercy machine. An agent in Hollywood has been trying to sell it. No luck. Why? Too controversial. CBS does no "theme" material anymore. God forbid they should attempt to deal with an issue like death. Or the right to die.

Maybe my proposal was poorly written. Maybe it was poorly structured. Non-dramatic. Dull. Lousy character development. Not enough suspense. Lacking in pathos. Or irony. Or. . . . But these weren't the reasons it was rejected. Not one producer made such criticisms.

Too controversial. Too substantive. Too meaningful.

I'll take Jesse Helms every time. He at least assumes that creative art is supposed to be meaningful.

Roger

May 12

Dear Rob,

I just got back from another quick trip to Indianapolis. I'm very big there. Not as a writer, of course. How could I be, with their scarcity of bookstores? Not that I would be if they suddenly had a surfeit, a plethora, a plague of bookstores. I was asked to give another lecture on Parkinson's disease. This one was again sponsored by Sandoz, the people who distribute Eldepryl for Mylan. You remember Mylan. You sold their stock as the result of insider information I gave to you. Ivan Boesky has nothing on us. Except a few hundred million dollars.

I gave a talk to a group of family practitioners. What could I say? The PSG results are still clothed in secrecy. We cannot give out the results or rather the non-results until the paper finally comes out. And the paper is still being written. So all we have to go on are the results we published previously in the *NEJM*. I can't disclose the real truth, the fact that Landau was right. No insider information for them.

Why not?

We have to wait until our results are peer reviewed. And published. The former is what science is all about. The latter? P.R. But I can't go on selling a drug for an effect it doesn't have. I know I'm not selling the drug. I'm giving a scientific talk sponsored by a drug company. But what happens to science if I know a hypothesis was not supported and I have to say that it was?

So what could I say about Eldepryl? That it has a therapeutic effect? Yes. That it has a protective effect? Six months ago I knew what to say. I still do. Only it's different. So I toned it down. Fortunately the title of my talk was wonderfully vague. "An Update on Parkinson's Disease." I talked mostly about how to make the diagnosis and the use of other drugs and where we stand on implants.

And fortunately no one asked me about Landau's letters. Their mothers, I suppose, do not subscribe to *Neurology*.

Otherwise the trip was as uneventful as expected. I still could not find a bookstore. No new plethora. If there is a plague on the houses or malls of Indianapolis, it is not made up of bookstores. I did count six more video stores and two more Pizza Huts. Another Venture. A Wal-Mart in progress. One less Kentucky Fried Chicken. Excuse me, KFC. Fried is out. *Out.* As out as real books, as novels. Not as typed word assemblages.

Bill Brashler said it best. "We are harpsichordists, plain and simple," he said to me. "Anachronisms."

"We could try a screenplay or two," I suggested.

"We are harpsichordists. We don't double on the piano forte."

"But I do like Beethoven," I sighed.

Roger

May 13

Dear Rob,

There has been a flurry of activity on the Bloom front. The good ol' *Bloom vs. Kramer et al.* And that flurry has involved us all: Bloom, Kramer, et al. I know I've not kept you abreast. No cc:s on the bottom of long letters. No copies of memos. No Xeroxes of subpoenas. Nothing. Sheer negligence on my part. Unfair to you. And our reading public. Correction, my reading public. I learned that switch from Burt Shapiro. My book. My public. And why have you been left out? It's virtually all been done over the phone. And, remember, there is no way to collect phone calls. Or send copies of them. I did warn you of that problem. More than once. I make far more than 7.6 phone calls a day. Dodgson

246

was lazy, unproductive, a piker. Hell, I make 7.6 long distance calls a day. How else could AT&T stay in business? And MCI? And Sprint?

It all began about three weeks ago with an offer from Marvelous Marty Bloom via Harriet Steinfeldt to me via Randall Jackson and to Sharp Books by way of Joe Tinker to settle the suit. The offer was like a Bloom fast ball. Hard to resist. For how much was he willing to settle? $10,000.

Not much for a wrongful death. It comes out to $125 per inning for his entire major league career. In 1950 that would have been okay. Twenty-five grand for two hundred innings. Pretty good in fact. Up there with the likes of Warren Spahn. With the best of them. But by today's standards that's terrible. Some guys get that much for each pitch. But Marty last pitched in '51. So today's inflated salary structure does not apply to him.

When Jackson called me, I told him that we should offer $7,500 or one hundred dollars per inning. He was no Warren Spahn. Jackson missed that one. And that we should split it 50-50. One half from me. One half from Sharp Books. That became the offer. And after a series of calls, Bloom accepted it.

So did Burt Shapiro. Sort of. He demanded that I still had to pay all their legal fees. How much was that? $23,000 plus change. That was $375 per inning. Three times what Bloom got. More than Spahn made until the '60s. In their terms, it was $250 per hour. They are working at today's prices after all.

I balked. They were piggybacking on my lawyer. He was doing the work and he hadn't worked that many hours. Besides, they still owed me royalties. Both me and my agent.

How much? Jackson asked me.

I had no idea. They had never sent me any detailed royalty statements.

He'd take care of that. He did. And in less than a day, complete royalty statements appeared by the magic of fax. I read them. They made very interesting reading. According to their own statement, Sharp Books owed me some $15,000 in royalties. And I owed them $23,000 for legal fees. More faxes. More phone calls.

In the end, we compromised. I'm getting one half of my royalties and we're going to call it even. *Bloom vs. Kramer et al.* is history. Settled. Gone. But not forgotten. Not if I can help it.

Roger

May 20

Dear Rob,

I've been caught again. For the third time. I guess that means I'm out. No, that it's out. Gone. History. And it's one of my favorite stories. It's the story of one of the founding fathers of American neurology, William Alexander Hammond, a great figure in the history of American neurology and American medicine as a whole.

What did he do, you ask. I'll tell you. He became Surgeon General during the Civil War. As such, he reorganized the Army Medical Corps into an efficient, lifesaving unit. He set up the world's first neurologic hospital. He founded one of the first pathology services, the Armed Forces Institute of Pathology. He wrote the first American textbook of neurology. He described a "new" movement disorder, athetosis.

Athetosis means "without posture" and that term was invented by Hammond to describe the inability of a patient of his who had recovered from a stroke to hold his hand in a stable, fixed posture because of continuous, slow, spontaneous movements of the fingers, thumb, hand, and wrist. Athetosis. Without posture. Other neurologists claimed that this was not a specific disorder, but in the end Hammond has been vindicated. Athetosis exists. It is a specific form of abnormal movements seen following strokes, or as part of the brain damage in cerebral palsy. But it is uncommon.

And he was court-martialed, found guilty of malfeasance, and cashiered out of the service. He became the only Surgeon General to have been court-martialed and the only one to be found guilty and be given a dishonorable discharge.

But he rose from the ashes. The phoenix of American neurology. He became a successful neurologist in New York, wrote his textbook, helped found the American Neurologic Association, and got the Senate to reopen his court-martial case and the Senate overturned his conviction.

Vindication.

It had been dirty politics. Secretary of War Stanton had played dirty pool. I did all the research and wrote up the story clothed in the story of a patient I'd seen with athetosis and put it into *Toscanini's Miscue*. So what happened? It was rejected by the editors and deleted from the book. The world got *Toscanini* sans *The Surgeon General*.

But I still liked the story. I still do. I had other options. A new book. A new publisher. A new editor. I'd try again. So I touched it up a bit and

248

slid it into *The Expert Witness*. New publisher. New editor. Same result. Was someone telling me something? Strike two.

I was frustrated, but not without recourse. I am at work on yet another book. I am at the earliest stage. Preparing a treatment for my agent. You remember him. He'll then submit it. To some other publisher, with some other new editor. You guessed it. So I put *The Surgeon General* into my latest book proposal.

Strike three. My agent deleted it. It's out. Gone but not forgotten. I suspect I'll submit it to *MD*. I'm sure they'll like it. It is a medical publication. Back to batting 1.000.

The poem, by the way, was written by a reporter named Burt Leston Taylor. The dinosaur poem. How did I find out? I wrote to Stephen Jay Gould. Always go to the best source. I told him my painful foot-moving toes story and asked him.

I also told him my amphioxus story. I'll tell that one to you now.

"Why," a student once asked me, "does the left side of the brain control the right side of the body?

"Because," I explained, "the parietal eye of early amphibians had a lens."

I could tell that she had not grasped the full meaning of my answer, so I elucidated it.

On that long trip from amphioxus to man, one stage was the amphibians. Many amphibians developed a single extra eye in the top of the head. This eye was above the parietal lobes and is occasionally called the parietal eye, athough it is more often called the pineal eye because it served to transmit signals to the pineal area of the brain. The pineal eye has a lens, and it's the lens that makes all the difference.

If an object, say some insect the amphibian would love to eat, moves from left to right, the image on the retina of the pineal eye also moves. If there were no lens, the image would move in the same direction. If there is a lens, however, the image moves the other way, to the left. The fly is now on the right. And the image is on the left side of the pineal retina and the left half of the brain. And the amphibian still wants to eat that fly.

To eat it, he must catch it; to catch it, he must see it. So as the fly moves farther to the right, he must turn his eye by lowering the right side. A muscle on the right side of the head must pull that lens down. But the sensation to trigger that movement is in the left brain. So the left brain has to send a nerve out to that muscle on the other side of the skull—from left to right. That phenomenon is called decussation, or crossing of nerve fibers, and it all started with the amphibians, the amphibians and God. Unfortunately, I misspelled amphioxus. Gould, forgive me.

Roger

Enclosure. N.B. Enclosure deleted by agent prior to submission.

May 26

Dear Rob,

I was in Geneva last weekend. Just for two days. I went to see Fred Gould. What a disaster! His friend, Michel Adler, picked me up at the airport. He's known Fred since they went to school together in Alexandria. He warned me that our friend was not doing well. That turned out to be a masterpiece of understatement. Sort of like saying that the victims of the St. Valentine's Day Massacre had had better days. A real Chicago metaphor. Or was that a simile?

We got to the house, a large house, on the outskirts, on the lake, and Mr. Adler asked me to wait in Fred's office. "Maybe we should have accepted him in our program," I said to myself as I waited there to see him. I knew we couldn't have. We had been doing research. A study. Not supplying a service. Research. *Research. Science.* How bad was he?

The office was elegant. What had I expected? Even the art was elegant. I sat there and stared at the de Chirico over the small couch opposite his desk. You must know de Chirico. Everyone does. The only surrealist to paint surrealistic paintings before Tzara invented surrealism. Or Breton. Or Duchamp. Or whoever did. I was never sure. He was the grand Dada who came before Dada. It was one of de Chirico's metaphysical pictures, one of the PITTURA METAFISICA. That was what de Chirico was famous for. You must have seen reproductions of them. I had seen this one before. Or had I? I knew the title, *The Disquieting Muses*. And the date, 1917. It's one of the handful of works that had made him one of the heroes of surrealism. His picture fit my mood perfectly. Disquiet in its most silent and most anguished state. Research, not patient care. It was research.

No artist had ever had a more brilliant beginning to a career. De Chirico had catapulted to fame as quickly as Sandalio Garcia. Nor had any artist that I could recall ever had a more complete fall from grace.

He went from the great genius of the PITTURA METAFISICA to become the world's first neoclassicist. The jigsaw puzzle components assembled in his metaphysical cityscapes, those arcades, those quiet towers, the trains, the silent statues, the menacing mannequins, the still piazzas and the shadows, those shadows of all shadows, all disappeared to be replaced by prancing horses and broken Ionic columns. Or were they Doric? Or Corinthian? A harbinger of things to come. A call to the return of classicism. A clarion call answered only by Walt Disney in his twelve minute version of Beethoven's *Pastoral* symphony. What, I wondered, would Garcia do next?

After two decades of unsuccessfully pursuing a lonely course as the world's premiere neoclassicist, de Chirico was in all the art books but only for his early, surrealistic works. The rest of his art was being totally ignored. He was painting pictures that no one wanted to buy. It was not the neoclassical ones that were in those art books. It was only his old metaphysical pictures. They had become a part of art history. He was a classic. His name was a household word. In some circles. And his art was sought after by the best museums and the richest collectors. And he couldn't make a living. There had to be something he could do. There was. The answer was obvious. Any Dadaist would have done the same thing. He created "later" versions of all his famous pictures. The ones that were in all the art books and all the museums. "Later versions" of his own pictures. Critics consider that phrase to be a euphemism for late forgeries. But they were self-forgeries, the same image repainted by the same hand complete with the same date: 1917. So what if they were really painted in 1947 or 1957 or 1967? Three out of four of the numbers are right. Same image. Same painter. Same date on the canvas. That's three. Painted some other time. Big deal. Three for four. .750. A very respectable batting average. At least as reliable as most expert attributions of Rembrandt. Or any other great artist. There are at least eighteen different versions of *The Disquieting Muses*, all dated 1917 and all but one done between 1945 and 1962. At least one is in a major U.S. museum. And one is in Fred's office. And I was staring at it.

The critics have all assailed de Chirico unmercifully. They have been more critical of him than I have been of Garcia. And why? He was a forger. He somehow forged his own works. Is that really possible? All he forged were the dates. And does a work of art have less meaning if the date is different? Less beauty? Less truth? It's not as if he reported only two patients when he operated on closer to a dozen, and two of them had already died.

Why did de Chirico do it? What a question. For money. Who in Italy in 1945 didn't need money? But was that his only motive? Why not for revenge? Revenge on the modernist critics who praised his early works and panned what he thought were his more mature works, his real masterpieces? Revenge on the collectors who bought the former and not the latter? What did they know? Not what he knew; that his later works were better, greater, truly classics.

Or glory? To share in his own glory? What glory is there in painting works that don't sell? It is like writing plays no one produces. Or writing books no one is willing to publish. Self-fulfilling? Give me a break. One cannot really survive on the reflected glory of things you did in a past lifetime.

That I understand. Some of the research I did twenty years ago was damn good. On the cutting edge. Pace-setting. So what? That is not where I am now. Or who I am.

Why did de Chirico do it? If you had asked him, his answer would have been, "Why did I do what?" The art was in him and in his creation of it, not in the date on the lower right-hand corner. Art is never in the date.

Why did Garcia do what he did?

That, my friend, is a more complicated issue. Was it the money? The fame? The glory? In Mexico he is a national hero. Their only medical star. Superstar. And we all think we need superstars. The big leagues. TV. Countries. All of us. For the sake of science? Or all of the above?

Or he may be like de Chirico. If you asked him "why?" he'd answer, "what?" He is not a scientist. He's a surgeon out of his league. He may well think that he did everything as it should have been done.

After half an hour of waiting I was finally ushered into Fred Gould's bedroom. He was seated in a chair, an overstuffed chair, next to his hospital type bed. Seated. Tied in with a cloth belt.

Tied into his chair!

I examined him. Fred had had a major stroke. Most of his right frontal lobe had been destroyed. And some of the left. He was confused. He babbled like a bewildered three-year-old. A rather inarticulate, bewildered three-year-old. His left arm was all but useless. He had to be fed. And held up to walk. When had this happened?

The day after surgery, I was told. A surgical complication. A stroke caused by the operation. I looked at the CAT scans. The areas of damage were frightening.

Fred Gould was as far from a surgical success as a patient could be. He was neither better nor "junger," no matter what anyone said. But Garcia had said that all of his patients were better. *All.* All were better. I'd rather be worse.

To hell with science, we should have operated on Fred. He was my patient. My patient. Not Garcia's. *Mine!*

Fred will need a gastrostomy or some other sort of feeding tube or he will choke and get pneumonia and that will be that. Perhaps he'd be better off without.

"He only went because of you," Michel told me.

"I know. We turned him down," I said. "I had no choice," I added feebly.

"Not just that."

"Not. . .?"

"He did not really trust the Mexican results but you told him your patients also improved."

"They did."

"And he needed to get better. He needed a miracle."

"None of my patients got that much better," I protested.

"He thought they did."

"I never said that."

"No, but he heard that."

I wondered if Fred had ever known when his de Chirico had been painted. He must have heard the stories. Had he had it checked out? Or had he preferred to believe the date of 1917?

"Why," I asked, paraphrasing my son, "do people go somewhere where you can't even drink the water to get experimental surgery?"

Neither of us said a word. We both knew why.

I needed to get away, to spend some time all by myself. And there was something else I wanted to do in Geneva. There was a painting I wanted to see. Not a de Chirico, no matter what the real date. As far from a de Chirico as possible. A painting that is in no art history book and never will be, but one I wanted to see. And observe. Or absorb. It was a sort of pilgrimage I felt I had to make. Not to Lourdes. To the Petit Palais. In Geneva, the Petit Palais houses their Museum of Modern Art. Not of contemporary art. For they draw a line between the two. Modern does not mean recent, contemporary, but the art that saw itself as modern, as of the twentieth century, of the machine age, beginning with the Cubists and Futurists and Expressionists and ending when modernism no longer offered the answers, with the Second World War.

The Museum of Modern Art in Geneva has a painting by Max Jacob. I had read that obscure fact in an old book I was scanning, different meaning, in a used bookstore. A Max Jacob done in 1912 of a circus in Paris. It was not an art book. It was a book about the art community in Paris at the outbreak of World War One. Art and literature. Early Modernism. Picasso. Matisse. Modigliani. Apollinaire. Lipschitz. Braque. Derain. They all knew each other. It was a community. And it included Max Jacob. I had to see that painting.

So I walked there to see it. A modest-sized oil. Not very distinguished. Modern, yes. A bit too much influenced by Dufy and the Fauves. More than a bit. A lot of Derain in a way.

They had only one Picasso. A far better work. Done in '43. I couldn't look at it. The Max Jacob I studied.

I'm back home now and I'm listening to a Sox game. They're playing Baltimore. The Baltimore announcer is Rex Barney. He pitched for the old Dodgers. The real Dodgers. In Brooklyn. His career was a bit more distinguished than Marty Bloom's. Not much. He had great stuff but he had no control. He could not get his pitches into that little strike zone. His epitaph, "Had the strike zone been high and outside, he would have been in the Hall of Fame." Rex Barney.

Picture it. It's the World Series. The Dodgers and the Yankees. Barney is to pitch. The Yankees are heavily favored. Let's make it even. We'll make the strike zone high and outside.

Did baseball do that? Never. You can't change the rules. Not for Rex Barney. And not for Sandalio Garcia.

Roger

June

About five years after my role in this case had ended, I happened to run into the judge. He remembered me well. I had won the case for the government. I was impressed that he remembered me. What did he recall? I wondered. My succinct testimony on direct question? My clever response to cross-examination?

"Neither," he said.

"Neither?" I was puzzled. Perhaps it was both. He'd made the decision in favor of the government, and he'd said that I'd won the case. What did he recall? What had swayed him?

"Those pants!" he said.

"My pants?"

"Any expert who had guts enough to testify in pants like that had to be right."

"My pants?" I repeated.

"And that horrible red jacket."

Harold L. Klawans
Trials of an Expert Witness

June 1

Dear Rob,

It looks as if Freud may well have been right after all. Certainly not about Anna O. Nor Oedipus. Nor penis envy. Nor incest as wish fulfillment, but about cerebral palsy. And his being right should warm the cockles of every obstetrician in the United States. Or, if not, at least those of the insurers of every obstetrician in the United States. Not a bad accomplishment, considering that most of them won't even pay analysts' bills.

It's the old Little–Freud controversy, part of the history of neurology. Freud, you recall, began life as a neurologist. Little didn't. He began life and ended it as an orthopod. Little may have been as much the founder of modern orthopedics as Freud was the founder of modern psychiatry. Or vice versa. If not, more so. In 1861 Little presented a paper on cerebral palsy to the Obstetrical Society of London. Up to then, the entire concept of cerebral palsy was a quagmire. Botany without Linnaeus. It was Little who systematized our thinking on cerebral palsy and it was Little who suggested that abnormal delivery, difficult labor, premature birth, and lack of oxygen during birth—that whole process—was the event that led to cerebral palsy.

And lawsuits. But those only came later. Or more recently, to put it into our perspective. If cerebral palsy is due to something that went wrong during labor, then the obstetrician should have prevented it. It's his fault. Or hers. Sue the SOB.

Not so, said Freud. That was back in 1891. Freud did not believe that asphyxia neonatorum, loss of oxygen of the newborn, was the cause of cerebral palsy. Freud, before he invented psychoanalysis, was a neuropathologist and a child neurologist before there were pediatric neurologists. He was even Director of Neurology at the Institute of Children's Diseases in Vienna. And he wrote a book on cerebral palsy.

And what did he write? That the relationship between asphyxia neonatorum and cerebral palsy was far from proven. Look at what Little himself had said: Most apparently stillborn infants, infants not breathing at all, if saved, recover unharmed. And most cases of cerebral palsy have no such history.

And then Freud made his key remark, a comment that was more succinct than his description of castration anxiety: "One has to consider that the anomaly of the birth process, rather than being the causal etiological factor, may itself be the consequence of the real prenatal etiology." In other words, the abnormal birth process was a result of fetal abnormality, not a cause of anything.

Freud, unfortunately for those interested in cerebral palsy, carried his argument no further. After he published this book, Freud's interest in hypnosis and hysteria led him away from child neurology and on to the analysis of dreams. As a result, Little's ideas concerning perinatal asphyxia as the cause of cerebral palsy remained largely unchallenged. Cerebral palsy and birth asphyxia went hand in hand. Little's theory of a one-to-one relationship between perinatal asphyxia and cerebral palsy was believed for many years, by doctors, lawyers, and juries. Look at all those lawsuits and the huge judgments. To say nothing of those high insurance rates. But who was right?

Freud. Despite improved obstetrical technique, despite better monitoring, despite more Caesarean sections, the rate of cerebral palsy remains pretty much unchanged. It's the number of lawsuits that has gone up, not the incidence of cerebral palsy. It's just that the former makes you believe the latter. But Freud was right. Most kids with cerebral palsy never had any birth asphyxia. No asphyxia neonatorum.

Who cares if he was right about Anna O.? Or Alma Mahler? Or the wolf man? Just think, if Freud had stuck to neurology, your malpractice insurance rates would be a lot lower. But he didn't. He followed his own star. No wonder Freud bashing is in.

Roger

June 8

Dear Rob,

Garcia is now into using fetal implants to cure Parkinson's disease. And all this time I thought adrenal implants did that. Silly me. And made the patients younger, too.

How do I know? Let me count the ways.

Rumors. He is a big believer in the word of mouth. As well he should be. It has generated both fame and fortune for him. Fortune in the guise of patients. Patients who are clamoring for his help. Patients with money.

And news stories. I read about his new venture in the *Chicago Tribune*. And the *New York Times*. And countless other papers. In cut out clippings sent to me by patients, relatives of patients, friends of patients, surviving spouses and children of patients who have died, what have you, from around the country. As far as I could tell, he got more coverage than the Nobel Prize in medicine. Certainly far more than the Nobel Prize in literature. To say nothing of the National Book Award. Which is what most of these papers say about it. Name this year's Nobel Prize winner in medicine. Or in literature.

But I know even more. I know the facts. Not just rumors. Not a news flash. But hard scientific data. Or as hard and scientific as one can expect from Garcia. Which may make it less hard than the number of copies of any best-seller in print. Much less hard than the actual number sold.

My knowledge has resulted from a combination of all of the above. Rumors. News. Data. In that chronologic order. Just like before. But there is one big difference, the significance of which is not subtle. This time the *New England Journal of Medicine* rejected his article. How do I know that? I was one of the experts who was asked to review it. Why? I'm sure they are well aware of my criticism of them for having said nothing when the facts about Garcia and his first set of results became known.

What did I say in my review?

Guess!

But the *New England Journal of Medicine* will be able to fill their pages without Garcia and still be in the forefront of the implant story. We sent them our paper and they are going to publish it. It's the results on our dozen patients plus patients from Florida and Kansas. We all followed the same protocol, so we grouped our results on a total of sixteen patients. And we left no one out. All of our patients showed some degree of improvement. The procedure helped. It did something for them.

But there were no cures. No miracles. We all got older and wiser. We are still following our patients and will report on them from time to time, but that part of my life is over now.

Roger

June 11

Dear Rob,

So you have also been rereading my letters to you. I haven't reread yours. I can't publish them. Thus, mine must stand alone. Yes, Tinker, Evers, and Chance are all in the Hall of Fame. They are the only double play combination to make it there. Deservedly so. Harry Steinfeldt was the third baseman for those Cubs teams. He is not in the Hall. Deservedly so. What choice did I have? I had to change the names of the real lawyers. Or the real names of the lawyers. They are all dead. Tinker, Evers, and Chance, I mean. I am not the only one who has appropriated their names. Evers' nickname was "The Crab." So when Bill Brashler decided to write a series of mysteries set in ball parks he wrote under the name "Crabbe Evers." He never even considered Marty Bloom. I would have used Jake Fox, as in Jacob Nelson Fox, the real name of Nellie Fox. Not in the Hall—a true tragic injustice. Or maybe Ken Keltner. He was the third baseman for the Indians. In 1941 he. . . .

By the way, *MD* loved "The Court-Martial of the Surgeon General." They loved it so much that they bought it. And I do mean bought it, for real money. And will publish it. It will see the light of day.

David stopped by. I told him about my success, trying to steer the conversation over to short works, individual short stories. Mine. His. I still have not read one of his. We drifted on to other subjects.

I have decided, by the way, that being a screenwriter is not the answer. Why do I say that? Why, when people who once read now universally watch instead? When every mall has two video outlets and no bookstores? I learned it from a video. Who says I'm out of date? From a videotape I rented. If you won't tell anyone, I won't. Not even David. The scene was in *Romancing the Stone*. The heroine, a writer of romance novels, and the rough and tumble hero, out of Sam Spade and Mike Hammer, find their way into the home base of some second-rate Colombian cocaine war lord. They are surrounded by cutthroats with guns. All pointed at them.

"Write your way out of this, Joan Wilder," he says.

"Joan Wilder," the drug lord says. "The writer?"

"Yes."

"I have all your books. I read them to the boys each Saturday night."

The writer's fantasy come true. Recognition in the middle of nowhere. More than mere recognition. Far more. And it was written by screenwriters. It's undoubtedly their fantasy, too. To be real writers. To write novels. Novels read around the world. Not screenplays, dissected by others and oft left on the cutting room floor. So much for the great American screenplay.

I don't even know who wrote that screenplay. How do you like that?

Roger

June 14

Dear Rob,

Yesterday I spent much of the day bumming around used bookstores. They are, in general, much more fun to wander through than new bookstores. Certainly than a Crown or a Waldenbooks. Try to find something out of the ordinary in one of them. I know they save you money on bestsellers, but there are still some of us who read books that aren't blockbusters.

Do you know how they make their money? Those book discounters? I hate to call them bookstores. We just don't have the right word for them. We do differentiate a fast-food franchise from a real restaurant, but a bookstore is a bookstore is a bookstore. Perhaps that's the phrase we need, fast bookstore. If the book doesn't sell fast, you have to look somewhere else.

So how do they clean up? Not on the best-sellers. Those have a very narrow margin of profit. They are not loss leaders, but close. They are the come-on that brings you in the door and right smack up to the publisher's remainders. Right up front. Published at $19.95, yours for only $5.95. What a bargain!

Their cost is $1.99 at the most. No one ever pays the publisher more than ten percent for a remainder and if you buy in big volume, you can get them for less. Say, $1.50. That makes their markup three hundred percent. Not a bad profit margin. And if they don't sell at $5.95, you can make a real sacrifice and cut the price to $4.50, leaving a markup of merely two hundred percent.

What a bargain! What a sacrifice! They're giving them away.

And on those art books, the markup is even greater. It's a business. But it has very little to do with literature. So I spend my free time crawling around the stacks in the used bookstores on Clark Street and Lincoln Avenue. It's not like Charing Cross Road used to be, but then neither is Charing Cross Road. And it's a lot closer than London.

I always go with a purpose, an excuse. A quest. My own Holy Grail, to be sought out. A late twentieth century Parsifal, without benefit of either Richard Wagner or Hermann Levi. So I went yesterday on that eternal search, that quest of all quests. You guessed it. I was looking for a book by Jen Peter Jacobsen. Rilke's hero. His Holy Grail. Not just any book, *the* book. That book of books. Book as Holy Grail. Mine. Rilke's. Except Rilke owned a copy. He took it with him wherever he went. Well, I, too, need a copy to read once and find out what all the fuss was about.

I struck out. It was like looking for memorabilia of Marty Bloom. And we never got to call a single one of those dealers to act as an expert witness. Do they have any Rex Barney cards? I used to have one. Déjà vu all over again. But I found some treasures. I always do. What do I consider treasures? A good question. Not an old Marty Bloom card. Not even an old Nellie Fox card.

Max Jacob. Any book by Max Jacob. Any book at all. I've mentioned him to you before. Last month I visited his painting in the Petit Palais in Geneva. Not his only painting, but the only one I have ever seen. The only one that I know still exists to be seen. There should be others. And books of his. There have to be. Max Jacob was the first modern French poet, a surrealist before his time. Friend of Picasso and Apollinaire before they were Picasso and Apollinaire, so to speak. A voice of Paris before the Great War, before the Jazz age, before Hemingway, Fitzgerald, and the invasion of expatriates. Jacob, who died of pneumonia in a cattle car on the way to the concentration camp at Drancy.

I found a book of his prose. Not much of a coincidence. Jacob was filed right there on the shelf that had nothing by Jacobsen. But, of course, it doesn't take very long to get through the J's. So I invaded other letters. And got other books.

Ben Hecht. Chicago writer. Worked as a columnist for a newspaper here in the teens and twenties. Wrote several successful plays. One classic, *The Front Page*. Coauthored with Charles MacArthur, one-time lover of Dorothy Parker of quip fame. Hecht gave up being a journalist in Chicago and went to Hollywood and wrote screenplays, even worked on *Gone With the Wind*. I bought a collection of his Chicago columns. And some Cocteau. And Cavetti. And Max Frisch. And as many copies of *Jerusalem Plot* as I could find.

Why? I'm out. Not sold out. I don't sell them. No one buys them. I'm given out. I don't have any copies left. And if I'm ever to sell the reprint rights, I'll need copies to send away to prospective publishers.

I found four. But no Jacobsen. Not a single copy. More copies of *From Here to Eternity* than you'd ever be able to read. Lots of P.D. James. Hundreds. Thousands. Did any great poet ever look upon her as his Holy Grail?

When *Sins of Omission* had just been published, I first saw a copy of it in a bookstore on a table of new books. New arrivals. Not publisher's remainders. This was a real bookstore. The front featured new arrivals. The store had a whole stack of my book. An entire stack of *Sins of Omission*. There they were right next to a stack of the newest book by Alan Paton, the South African writer. If you haven't read *Cry, the Beloved Country*, run, do not walk, to a real bookstore and get a copy. New or used. In any condition. You will probably not find one at your local Crown. Nor Waldenbooks. Try a real bookstore. There must be one near you.

I couldn't believe it. There I was, right next to Alan Paton. A juxtaposition I could not fathom. What justice was there in that? I said something to the owner.

"You are right," he said. "I've already sold a dozen copies of your book. I'll be lucky to sell one of his."

I bought two. One I gave to David.

If you run into any Jacobsen while getting *Cry*, buy it for me. And all the copies of *Jerusalem Plot* you can find. And of course get yourself copies of *Murder in Wrigley Field* and *Bleeding Dodger Blue* and *Murderers' Row*. You'll find them under E for Evers, not B for Brashler.

Roger

June 16

Dear Rob,

Today is Bloomsday, the eighteen-hour-long day during which the hero of Joyce's *Ulysses* wandered the streets of the city of Dublin. Literature's first Jewish hero. Hemingway does start *The Sun Also Rises* by introducing Robert Cohen. Cohen is not a hero. Or was he? He was the first Jew in Western literature who hit back.

Well, Bloom, the Bloom of *Ulysses*, Joyce's Bloom, not my Bloom, not Martin Bloom, but the real Bloom, Leopold Bloom, was created to be the first anti-hero. The first Jewish anti-hero. Recreating myth. Doing battle not with sirens or cyclopses, but with the ordinary commonplace issues of everyday life. The twentieth century at work and play.

Leopold Bloom. On June 16, 1904. In Joyce's Dublin. Bloomsday.

No. I have not changed my mind about *Ulysses*. The book is too diffi-cult, too convoluted, too complex. Joyce tried to do too much. To recre-ate myths. To restructure the novel, to reconstruct language, to self-con-sciously create modern literature. Modern is a word I've always distrust-ed. That mistrust comes from my first trip to Europe. That was in the summer of '58. So long ago. I and my three college roommates spent ten weeks driving through Europe.

How long ago was that? So long ago that four roommates meant four guys, none of whom were gay. Or knew they were gay. Or thought they might be. And any hotel called modern, *Hotel Moderne*, we learned was to be avoided like the plague. Moderne meant vintage 1914 and never remodeled. Modern in the sense of the Museum of Modern Art in Geneva. Is Max Jacob's *Circus* modern? Is early Picasso?

I cut my teeth on Joyce. *Portrait* and *Dubliners* and on Conrad and Eliot. Beckett, Gide, Camus, Hemingway, Faulkner. They all came later. But whenever I write, their spirits hang over me. Each morning as I get up and make my coffee, I, too, imagine a life measured out in coffee spoons. Or was it in coffee ladles? No matter.

But is a man to be judged solely by his lines? Even a poet?

A man is his poetry. And vice versa. It may not matter, in the end, if you cheat the IRS or cheat on your wife, but what does matter is whether you cheat on yourself. And it applies to writers more than sci-entists. You have to stand up and be counted on those few issues that matter. If the Germans seize Max Jacob, you have to stand up and be counted.

Eliot wanted us to believe that poetry had to do only with poetry. *The Waste Land* is about poetry. It is about its own creation. About the fate of European civilization. But not about politics. His politics didn't matter.

Like hell. Eliot was at best a reactionary, a great admirer of Charles Maurras. Maurras was a French Fascist before his time. Late in his life, Maurras was able to live out his Fascist fantasies. He was both a writer and a politician. He was the principle founder of Action Francaise, an ultra right-wing movement. The Godfathers of Le Pein. Maurras loved Mussolini. And Franco. And Marshall Pétain, Premiere of Vichy, France under the Nazis.

When the war was over, Maurras was tried for collaboration with the Nazis and sentenced to life in prison. The French didn't do that to many collaborators. There were not enough jails to hold them all.

Eliot would never have signed Cocteau's petition. No one would have bothered to ask him. He would have been too busy collaborating.

What makes Siegfried Sassoon, a minor poet, a gadfly at best, what makes him important is that he knew that politics mattered. Sending young men out to be killed for no real reason mattered. It was wrong. A tragedy. A reason for poetic protest. Protest that was far more important than a million *Waste Lands*. But who writes Ph.D. theses on Sassoon?

Auden, too, was brought up on Eliot. There should be no connection between politics and poetry. Poetry had to do with some sort of abstract truth, abstract beauty. The poet should be as detached as the scientist. Yet we are not detached. We can't be. Auden learned better. Did Eliot? He should have already known better.

Unlike Bloom's, my day today did not last eighteen hours. Closer to twelve. Including this letter. It was a day measured more in out-patient visits than in coffee spoons. One every fifteen minutes. An average day in the office. From 9:00 to 12:00 I saw twelve patients. From 1:00 to 5:00 another sixteen. Twenty-eight in all. What's the big deal? Lots of doctors see that many patients in a day.

Twenty-eight patients. Think about it, Rob. Not twenty-eight pelvic exams for routine Pap smears. Not a couple of dozen people coming in for routine physicals, routine check-ups, routine care. But twenty-eight people with significant neurologic disease, not mere aggravations, not headaches, not low back pain. Not dizziness. Thank God.

Real disease. Progressive disease. Parkinson's. Huntington's. Dystonia. Even a case of athetosis. Epilepsy. And a single patient with multiple sclerosis. I've been treating her for over twenty years. We're old friends. She's now in her seventies. She walks with a foot brace and uses a four-pronged cane. In the twenty years I've known her, she's had twenty attacks. They used to occur every nine months. Like clockwork.

Now they are farther apart. The last one was eighteen months ago.

"Why?" she asked me.

It was a good question. I tried to give her an answer. In MS, the immune system is for some reason attacking the nervous system. As we get older, the immune system wears down. MS becomes less active.

Her husband is also my patient. But only for eight years, although I've known him for twenty years. First as his wife's pillar of support and care-giver. Then he developed Parkinson's disease.

And then two strokes. One on the day he retired. He, too, has a foot brace and a four-pronged cane. And now he is more disabled than his wife. Care-giver has become care-receiver. They gave up their home and live in a retirement center. And now he has a new problem. Kaposi's sarcoma.

"Why?" he asked me. "Why?"

Because he is old and his immune system is failing.

And through this all I am to remain a detached scientist? Give me a break! That's not how I judge myself.

Roger

June 17

Dear Rob,

The Waitkus shooting took place on June 14, 1949. I've been hunting down all of the original information. Her name was Ruth Ann Steinhagen. She registered at the Edgewater Beach Hotel as "Ruth Ann Burns." She was nineteen years old. She ordered a couple of drinks and slipped the bellboy a few bucks to give a message to another guest in the same hotel. Eddie Waitkus. First baseman for the Philadelphia Phillies. Eddie was twenty-nine years old.

In due time, Eddie showed up at her room. Shortly thereafter, she shot him. He missed the rest of the season.

Ruth Ann Steinhagen was apparently obsessed by Waitkus. She had previously been equally obsessed by Alan Ladd and Franz Liszt. How's that for a peculiar lineup? An old double play combination: Ladd to Liszt to Waitkus. She'd been obsessed with Waitkus since she'd been sixteen.

According to the newspapers, she was diagnosed as having a "split personality" and sent off to a mental institution. It's unclear what they meant by "split personality." More likely schizophrenia than multiple personalities. That was before *All About Eve*. And *Sybil*. Split personalities, multiple personalities weren't in. Today they are. Not more common. Just in vogue. She remained institutionalized for three years. Sort of like Anna O.

Waitkus came back in time for the 1950 season. He played all 154 games. He got the Comeback Player of the Year award. The Phillies won the pennant and lost the World Series to the Yankees in four straight games. Waitkus got four hits in the Series.

The shooting took place in room number 1297-A. And Malamud's *The Natural* was based on Eddie Waitkus. Not Billy Jurges.

Roger

June 18

Dear Rob,

I'm sorry to hear that your mom died. It was not so long ago that my own mom died. 1986. She was 87. I thought she was 86, but she was a year older than she ever told us. She'd been born in 1899, not 1900, and had lied to us all these years. And stuffed away in her drawers were hand-dipped chocolate candies, which she had delivered to her once a month or so.

And in her medicine cabinet, the Seconal I had given her. We had an understanding, she and I. She never wanted to go into a hospital again. She had severe angina. She could hardly go out anymore. I would try to keep her at home and she'd do exactly what her doctor advised. And I gave her the Seconal, in case.

She never needed that. The bottle was unopened. Not so the hand-dipped chocolates. So much for her doctor's dietary instruction. But that's as it should be.

I guess you'll have to take out your own subscription to *Neurology*.

Roger

Letter to an Unknown Agent

Dear Unknown Agent:

I appreciate the fact that you are willing to consider representing me. Before we enter into any negotiations, you should have a complete understanding of my literary history.

My first book was published without any representation. I know that that is anathema to you, but it does happen sometimes. I had run into an old acquaintance who had published a book and he gave me the name of his publisher. I submitted my first novel to him based on this introduction. Not exactly over the transom. Or under the door. Or through the window. It was published in 1982 by Sharp Books. This novel, entitled *Sins of Omission*, was a Book-of-the-Month Club alternate selection. Paperback rights of that book were never sold. At least not by Sharp Books. Sharp then rejected my second novel, and eventually all rights for *Sins* were returned to me. At that point, I began searching for an agent and wound up with Hank Thompson. How did I pick him? Easy. He was a Mets fan. He had been a Giants fan before they moved to San Francisco. Maybe that should have told me something. Hank then sold the paperback rights for three novels, mass distribution, while retaining all secondary and foreign rights. These were: *The Brain Implant, Jerusalem Plot,* and the paperback of *Sins of Omission*. They are all now out of print and the copyright on all three has been returned to me. It should be noted that these were three related novels involving the same main character, Paul Richardson. They were, however, never sold as a series, at least not in the United States. Isn't it series that mystery publishers crave?

I have subsequently written one more Paul Richardson novel called *The Blind Observer*. This has yet to be sold anywhere.

As far as my non-fiction publications, these were all represented by Hank Thompson. The first of these was *Toscanini's Miscue*. The contract for this was negotiated in an elevator between me and Burt Shapiro, President of Sharp Books, who basically commissioned me on the spot to write the book. This book became a Literary Guild alternate selection and was later published in paperback by Bantam, and has now been sold in some eight or nine other countries. Hank's major contribution to my career came in the selling of the successor, *The Expert*

Witness. This was sold for a very hefty advance. It remains in print.
I am enclosing a précis of my newest project.

Sincerely,

Roger Kramer, M.D.

The Chicago Trilogy
by
Harold L. Klawans

This trilogy is a departure from standard, multivolume sagas. It intentionally employs a number of unities that are ordinarily not a part of the organization of such undertakings. The works invoke unities of time, place, person, and narrator. At the same time, they violate rules of unity as to style, format, and content. Rather than a set of consecutive novels chronologically and comprehensively telling the story of a single character over time, these books all occupy the same time frame and involve the same character, both as subject and as narrator. Each volume differs from the other two in relation to what the narrator allows to be included for the select audience for whom that volume was apparently intended. Each of the novels centers around a selected aspect of the life of the main character, Paul Richardson, a fifty-year-old physician-writer. All three books take place over the same twelve-month period of time, a single academic year at Paul's medical school, beginning on July first and ending on the next June thirtieth. Each of the books deals with a separate aspect of Paul Richardson's life. All three books are completely controlled by Paul, who is both character and narrator. In each, Richardson is making a conscious, highly selective attempt to pull together and make sense of a single aspect of his life, as if getting that straight is the single most important part of coming to terms with who he is. And why. In the same way that each book deals with separate aspects of his life, each is organized differently and presented in a different manner to the reader. The first is organized by months and the days of each month, the second by weeks, and the third by quarters of the year. In order to carry out the separateness and uniqueness of each year, the three books are stylistically independent. Each, of course, stands alone as any novel must, but each is directly related to the other two and the overall fabric of the trilogy is intertwined into what is, hopefully, a truly synergistic fashion. The one model for this trilogy is British playwright Alan Ayckbourn's three related plays—*The Norman Conquests*. These three plays revolve around everything that happens to Norman over a single weekend. The plays are artificially divided such that each play consists of only those scenes that occur in a single room over that weekend. We thus see three separate stories and, of course, a fourth tale that arises from having seen all three. Each play stands alone and can be done as a single evening's entertainment, but the whole is enriched over that which is derived from each of the parts.

The first book, tentatively titled *On the Cutting Edge—A Book of Months* is an epistolary novel comprised of letters from Paul Richardson to a physician whom he has not seen in almost thirty years. This physician was an intern with Paul when they spent a year together in the trenches learning how to be doctors. Or, as Paul puts it, "learning grace under fire." The other physician had initiated the interaction by writing to Paul and asking his advice in embarking on his own fledgling literary career. In a series of individually dated letters spread out over the year, Paul attempts to explicate his life as a physician/scientist and his life as a writer. Paul limits these letters to his professional life or, more correctly, to his two professional lives. Every effort is made to avoid the personal. It is the battle between the two cultures that must be resolved. Paul as scientist vs. Paul as artist. Paul as physician vs. Paul as writer. Scientific insight vs. literary insight. Creativity vs. creativity. Data vs. imagination. Paul delves into the contradictions, competitions, and interactions of these two not quite so separate lives. This, then, is the fabric of these letters and the enigma that Paul must resolve as he wavers on the cutting edge between two worlds.

The second novel is tentatively titled *The Play's the Thing—A Weekly Reading*. Much like the first book, this novel is also triggered by a figure from Paul Richardson's past. This, however, is a person who had a major emotional impact on Paul's life, a woman who was his lover almost two decades earlier. She is now going blind from a progressive neurologic disease. The book will be organized as a series of audiotapes sent each Sunday by Paul to this woman; hence the title, *A Weekly Reading*. These readings center both on Paul's relationship to this woman, past and present, and its effect on both his literary works and his scientific works. This effect is one that Paul only comes to understand during the course of the year and stands out in stark contrast to the picture he has been painting in his letters of the detached scientist and writer.

The third novel, entitled *A Novel Approach—Four Quarterly Reports*, consists of the novel that Paul writes during this single year. The novel has four sections, one of which is completed during each quarter of the year and each of which is presented from the perspective of a different character. Not really *The Sound and the Fury* revisited, but a sequential story told in sequence by four participants. The novel, of course, stands on its own two feet as an independent novel, and relates to Paul's alter ego coming to terms with his personal life and attempting to integrate his personal life with his professional life. It is the story of a year-long, complicated affair between a fifty-year-old professor at a medical school in Chicago and a medical student who is half his age. The novel, as part of the trilogy, is enriched by a greater knowledge of how it was created, why it was created, and how it reflects upon its creator and thus gives meaning to and derives meaning from the other two works. For it is the novelization of Paul's personal life during a year. That year? Perhaps.

June 25

Dear Rob,

Believe it or not, David found a copy of *Niels Lyhne* by Jens Peter Jacobsen. How could I have ever doubted that he would? Actually, he found two copies. Not just two copies, but copies of two different translations. One he is now reading. The other he lent to me. It was done by someone named Tijna Nunnally. The book was published in 1990 by Fjord Press in Seattle, Washington. Not exactly Random House. But any port in a storm. No pun intended.

At the end of the book, there is a list of other translations published by Fjord Press, books by such authors as Hans Scherfig *(Stolen Spring)* and Klauss Rifbjerg *(Witness to the Future)*. I'd never heard of any of them. Neither the books nor the authors, but then again I'd never heard of Jacobsen either. I'd ask David about them, but then he would get the books and then I'd have to read them. I'm certain they are all important writers who wrote important books that are well worth reading. But I'm busy. I have to read *Niels Lyhne*. In two different translations yet.

According to the information on the fly leaf, the novel is the story of a young man's existential struggle. It's all about the great issues of late nineteenth century existentialism—a nice anachronism, that. It's about romanticism and atheism and an artist caught between his reality and his dream. Sort of like being caught between medicine and literature.

Jacobsen, it seems, did not write very much. Two novels. One volume of short stories. A few poems. Yet everyone read him. The list of those who felt a debt to Jacobsen's work is impressive. Thomas Mann. August Strindberg. Jean Giraudoux. Herman Hesse. Henrik Ibsen. Even our old friend Sigmund Freud admired his work. So did James Joyce. And Stefan Zweig. And, of course, Rainer Maria Rilke. We must not forget Rilke. He's the one who got me into this.

The back fly leaf quoted Zweig. "*Niels Lyhne*—how ardently, how passionately we loved this book in the first years of youthful awareness: it was the *Werther* of our generation. Countless times we read this melancholy biography, knew whole pages of it by heart, and the thin, worn volume accompanied us to school and late at night to bed; even today, when I look up some passages in it, I am at once able to write them down word for word from memory, because we had so often, so passionately absorbed those scenes into our lives."

One more thing. Jacobsen was a scientist, a botanist. He translated Darwin into Danish. A scientist and a poet. He, too, tried to lead a double life. Life with a wife and a mistress. But ill health, it said, made him choose. Science or literature. Wife or mistress. He deserted science. It was illness that forced a choice. Not a metaphysical crisis. Tuberculosis complete with coughing up blood. The same fate as Kafka. And Chekhov. And so many others. Not just literary characters, but their creators, too.

Perhaps my interest in Oscar Kokoschka is not entirely displaced. I am not, it seems, the first neurologist to have had an interest in him. After all, art and neurology do meet from time to time. In 1907, just at the outset of his fledgling career, Oscar Kokoschka traveled from Vienna to Switzerland to do a portrait of Auguste Forel. Forel was one of the founders of neurology. His biography is one of the sketches that make up a book with that title. In 1871 he wrote a paper in which he proposed that individual cells or neurons were the independent, functional units that made up the brain. The neuron theory of the brain, a pivotal advance. The word *neuron* was not coined for another twenty years.

In 1898 Forel retired and nine years later Kokoschka did his portrait. The family hated it and refused to pay for it. It didn't look like their father. Kokoschka made him look too old, too debilitated. It's now in a museum in Mannheim. In 1912 Forel had a stroke. His right side was paralyzed. At the age of sixty-four, he learned to write with his left hand. He died in 1931.

I got a call today from one of the neurologists who is collaborating with us on our implant research. By chance, our conversation turned to Garcia. He had visited Garcia in Mexico City. Back at the beginning.

"What," I asked, "did Garcia do before he got busy doing adrenal implants?"

"I thought you knew. He did septal resections for schizophrenia."

"That Hofer business?"

"Yes," he told me.

"But that never worked. No one else ever replicated that work. Nobody believes that that operation cures anybody."

"So, why should that have stopped him?"

"You knew that?"

"Yes. The first time I visited him, Garcia had a waiting room full of schizophrenics from all over Latin America. What a zoo."

"You knew that and still decided to do implants?"

"Did we have a choice?"

I'll let you answer that one.

Roger

P.S. I almost forgot. Michel Adler called. Fred Gould died.

June 26

Dear Rob,

Jeffrey Dahmer is dead. Murdered in prison by another prison inmate. Why did that fellow felon kill him? A voice told him to do it. The voice of God. Will we have another sanity hearing? Another parade of experts with only fifty percent interrater reliability?

He hears voices, ergo he must be insane. Are you certain of that? Was Saint Joan crazy? Where did she fit on the craziness scale? All her contemporaries gave her a zero. Not crazy at all. It was all a question of whether the voices came from God or the devil. Saint or heretic. But not crazy. Reread Shaw's introduction to *Saint Joan*. It's the best part of the play. But, as Groucho said, in a line most likely written by George S. Kaufman, "There ain't no sanity clause."

Why do I care about Hammond and his court-martial? I'll give you three guesses.

Bingo! You got it right on the first try. He was a writer, an author. Not just one of our first neurologists, but one of America's first physician-novelists. Our first neurologic novelist. Not our last. His novels were typical nineteenth century romances. I read two. I had all I could do to get through them. He was no Hemingway. In the last decade of his life, he became increasingly interested in religion, and his last novel, *The Son of Perdition*, centered around the life of Christ. This one is perhaps the least difficult to find. Marty Bloom baseball cards are easier to come by. Even you have one of those. If you really want a book by Hammond, I'll assign David to the case.

And you are, in a sense, right about Eliot. Not about *Murder in the Cathedral*. That is more like a sermon. Catholicism as High Art. High Mass as High Literature. Sassoon, too, converted. In 1957. As did Max Jacob, but both had better taste than to confuse dogma with art, creativity with ritual. But at least Eliot stole the ritual from a good source. And he did steal. He plagiarized. From Conan Doyle. *The Musgrave Ritual*.

Whose was it?

His who is gone.

Who shall have it?

He who shall come.

What was the month?

The sixth from the first.

Over the oak.

Where was the Shadow?

Under the elm.

How was it stepped?

North by ten, and by ten, east by five and by five, south by two and by two, west by one and by one, and so under.

What shall we give for it?

All that is ours.

Why should we give it?

For the sake of the Trust.

Eliot appropriated this ritual. He adopted it. He borrowed it. Had I done it, it would have been plagiarism. But Eliot is a certified genius. He could not possibly have borrowed anything from a hack physician-writer like Conan Doyle. Not from a story about Sherlock Holmes.

When the "similarity" between the sequence in *Murder in the Cathedral* (not quoted here as it is still under copyright) and the one in *The Musgrave Ritual* (quoted here as it is no longer under copyright) was finally noticed, and that took some time since Eliot and Sherlock Holmes are considered odd bedfellows by most, no one thought Eliot had borrowed from Conan Doyle. That would have been like Babe Ruth using Marty Bloom's bat. Worse. The mere thought is a sacrilege.

There must have been a common source, a little known Plantagenet ritual used by both Conan Doyle and Eliot. A common ancestry, appropriated independently by two men of letters. Eliot could not have borrowed from Conan Doyle. Not Eliot. Not from Conan Doyle.

But he did. And his use of Conan Doyle was, in Eliot's own words, deliberate and wholly conscious. When asked, he admitted to it. Outright borrowing. Plagiarism at its finest. But Eliot's poetry still matters. So must the man. Conan Doyle is listed in *The Concise Oxford Companion to English Literature*, but they make no mention of the fact that he was a physician. Hammond is not listed.

David came by. I had a question for him. A question about Doblin. Alfred Doblin. The German writer. Author of *Berlin Alexanderplatz*. That's his most famous book. Written in 1929. It may be the only big city novel in all of German literature. They do not have our tradition of muckrakers.

Did David know that Doblin was a physician?

No.

A neurologist?

"What is it with you guys? You neurologists? Isn't neurology enough for you?"

David always asks the right question. It's his job.

Roger

June 28

Dear Rob,

What a morning! At nine I got a call from Burt Shapiro of *Sins of Omission* and *Toscanini's Miscue* fame. Good ol' et al. My old friend. His parents were in town. His mother has Parkinson's disease and she was not doing well. Could I see her?

Why me?

"You're the best."

I could. I did. At 10:30. By noon Burt and I were having lunch. At his club. Talking like old friends. Friends who had been through a war together. I was talking about neurology. The brain. The role of evolution in neurologic disease. I told him my painful foot-moving toes story. I told him my amphibian-pineal eye story. No, I did not quote the dinosaur poem to him.

"That would make a good book," he said. "I'd like to publish it," he added.

Before dessert arrived we had a deal. Tentatively titled *Up from Amphioxus*. So once again I have a publisher. No thanks to my agent. I am no longer an outsider.

Over the weekend I tried rereading *Ulysses*. No, that's not true. I tried rescanning it. I made a terrible discovery. About Bloom. Leopold Bloom. Not Marty. I'm certain it is not an original discovery. It was only original to me. Bloom, Leopold, the Irish Jew. The Jewish Irishman. The outsider's outsider. The wandering Jew of Dublin.

But Bloom was not a Jew.

His mother wasn't Jewish. Ergo he was not a Jew. He lived on the outskirts of the Jewish community, neither Jew nor gentile. Neither proper Irish nor complete outsider. He could not have become Bar Mitzvah without first undergoing conversion. Bloom's knowledge of his heritage was limited; all but non-existent. When he read a Hebrew scroll, it came out, "Aleph, Bet, Ghimel, Daleth, Hagadah, Tephillim, Kosher, Yom Kippur, Hanukkah, Rosh Hashanah, B'nai B'rith, Bar Mitzvah, Mazzoth, Askenazim, Messhuggah, Talith." A gentile's list of Hebrew letters and words. A veritable word salad.

Did Joyce know?

He had to. That made his outsider even more of an outsider. A wanderer without a home. Who could never have a home. No matter what. Except with Max Jacob in that cattle car to Drancy.

Roger

June 30

Dear Rob,

A few confessions at the end. Nice and tidy. Are all the clinical tales I have told true? Are they real stories that happened to real people? In just the way I retold them? With just the names changed? To fictionalized names? Like Marty Bloom?

Of course not. I am both a scientist and a writer. An author. I know that there is a difference. But what is the difference?

One of my patients was published as a case report in *Neurology* in 1974. She became a landmark case. From patient to case. Note the transition. Later she became the subject of a clinical tale. I wrote to you about her before. See my letter of whatever date it was, if you kept it. I did. That was transition number two. Case back to patient. The same patient who had become the case report. But there was also another transition. She was never really a codified case. She was a patient and patients cannot become set in stone. Or print. Patients don't stay the same. They can't. They have to change. They continue to make transitions because they are not static objects. Nor am I. The patients I have treated for twenty years all know that I have changed. My view of them has changed. Their truth has evolved.

Are their stories true? Should they be? In that sense. Should there be a clinical file in my office under some other name that parallels each tale I have told? Did Melville ever see a white whale? What speech did Antony really make? What did he say? His words were buried with him. Too grandiose for you? Perhaps.

Was there a Josef K.? Or just his crime? Whatever that was. Yet the book has a ring of truth. A reality that superseded any history of life in a modern totalitarian state. Ever. And also preceded.

Medicine is not a compendium of lab tests and dosage schedules. And understanding the act of taking care of sick people has nothing to do with such facts. Genug! I'm tired.

David came by today. He is talking of retiring. He does that annually. His fantasy. To give up neuropsychiatry completely. To move to New York. To visit galleries and museums. To haunt the library. I've always thought his left wing tendencies, despite his claim to be an anarchist, came not from his father but from his identification with Marx, a man who actually spent his life in the reading room at the British Museum. He visited Marx's grave in London. A pilgrimage of sorts. So he is again talking of retiring. Two daughters are married. One, the youngest, a poet, has graduated. He can afford it.

Was he certain? After all, our professional income and lifestyle are seductive. His needs are few. Galleries are free. Museums cheap. Libraries cost nothing. All he buys is books. Mostly used books or remainders. Not at Crown, but by mail.

What would he miss?

The patients. The role of the seeker. The job of teasing out their narratives, of having people give you their lives, of asking you to help them reconstruct their stories. Of wanting to tell you everything so that they and you can make some sense out of it.

I agreed. That would be the hardest thing to put behind. That and the egosyntactic nature of our lives.

He knew what I meant. He is an expert in his field. Respected. Sought after. Lauded. No gallery owner will seek after him to come into his gallery and just look around. He will be just another visitor at the Met. Or the MOMA. Or even the Brooklyn Museum. And the libraries? Who knew that bearded man seated at a corner in the Readers' Room, same corner, every day, the one who needed a bath, that he was Karl Marx?

From a sort of fame to anonymity. From our world of acceptance to one of rejection. From being noticed to being ignored. The unkindest cut of all. But, I added, none of these are the real issue.

"What's the real issue," he asked, "if we retire?"

"Then we would have to be what we pretend to be."

He stopped. "You are right." He paused. "And profound." And he meant it. He didn't know I borrowed the essence from Vonnegut. He doesn't like Vonnegut.

So the questions, my friend, are obvious. Did you sign up for a workshop? Are you canceling one day of the office each week? Or are you, like too many of us, still satisfied with pretending?

Roger